Praise for Tanya Zuckerbrot, M.S., R.D., and

*The F-Factor Diet*

"*The F-Factor Diet* is packed with critical facts that form the foundation for a knowledge-based approach to lifestyle nutritional success. Tanya's scholarly approach is a gift that gives forever. Her contribution to preventive health care is immeasurable."
—Dr. Jerome Zacks, assistant clinical professor,
The Mount Sinai Medical Center

"Bravo for the F-Factor Diet. It is not a weight-loss diet but a lifestyle approach to eating healthy, satisfying, and delicious foods. It is not based on deprivation, but instead focuses on an expansive list of foods to create well-balanced meals and snacks that come together to comprise a healthy diet."
—Lisa Sasson, M.S., R.D., clinical associate professor,
New York University Department of Nutrition, Food Studies, and Public Health

"Tanya Zuckerbrot's approach to nutrition is sensible and based on science rather than fads. Under her guidance, my patients have significantly lowered their cholesterol, lost weight, and increased their chances of longevity."
—Ronald W. Galluccio, M.D.,
Eastside Medical and Cardiovascular Associates, New York

"A clear, easy-to-follow, and very informative book. Unlike many other diets, the F-Factor Diet promotes a healthful eating habit."
—Darlene Boytell-Perez, ARNP,
gastroenterology nurse practitioner

"The F-Factor Diet helped me lower my cholesterol and lose ninety pounds. Even dining out was never a problem. This is the best I have felt in years!"
—Brian Dennehy

"I would recommend *The F-Factor Diet* because that is a great book and a great way of eating . . . it works."
—Megyn Kelly, *NBC News*

# THE F-FACTOR DIET

## Discover the Secret to Permanent Weight Loss

TANYA ZUCKERBROT, M.S., R.D.

A TarcherPerigee Book

**tarcher**perigee

An imprint of Penguin Random House LLC
375 Hudson Street
New York, New York 10014

Most TarcherPerigee books are available at special quantity discounts for bulk purchase for sales promotions, premiums, fund-raising, and educational needs. Special books or book excerpts also can be created to fit specific needs. For details, write: SpecialMarkets@penguinrandomhouse.com.

ISBN 9780399533747 (paperback)

LIBRARY OF CONGRESS HAS CATALOGED THE G. P. PUTNAM'S SONS HARDCOVER AS FOLLOWS:
Zuckerbrot, Tanya.
The F-factor diet: discover the secret to permanent weight loss / Tanya Zuckerbrot.
p.        cm.
Includes index.
ISBN: 978-0-399-15412-6
1. High-fiber diet.   2. Reducing diets.   3. High-fiber diet—Recipes.
4. Reducing diets—Recipes.   I. Title.
RM237.6.Z83        2007        2006027010
613.2'5—dc22

Printed in the United States of America
30   29   28   27   26   25   24

Designed by Tanya Maiboroda

*To my other half, Anthony, and our children,*
*Tobey, Juliette, Olivia, Gabriel and Max.*
*Also for my Grandma Claire, who was always my biggest fan.*

# AUTHOR'S NOTE

I AM EXCITED to share with you the newly revised and updated *The F-Factor Diet*. Since its original release in 2006, countless people all over the world have relied on F-Factor to dramatically lose weight and improve their health without deprivation, denial, or hunger.

The "F" in *The F-Factor Diet* originally stood for one thing: fiber. Fiber is the indigestible part of carbohydrates. Fiber has numerous health benefits including lowering cholesterol, managing blood sugar levels, and building a healthy gut. But when it comes to weight loss, fiber's benefits put it into a league all its own. Fiber has zero calories, it adds bulk to foods (think larger portions with fewer calories), it revs metabolism, and it actually makes fat and calories in other foods disappear. That's right . . . the more fiber you eat, the more weight you lose.

Ten years after the original release of *The F-Factor Diet*, I've realized that the "F" in F-Factor stands for more than just "fiber." That F stands for "freedom." On F-Factor, you have the freedom to dine out for breakfast, lunch, or dinner, anywhere and everywhere. You have the freedom to eat carbs and even enjoy cocktails from Day 1. And since F-Factor doesn't require you to spend hours at the gym for results, you also get a lot of free time back. F-Factor isn't just about adding years to your life (which it does, as fiber has been linked to longevity!), but about adding life to your years.

This time around, F-Factor Diet's 3-Step Program is even easier and more enjoyable to follow, with more than twenty-five brand-new recipes, updated product recommendations, an increased net carb allowance, and two exciting *new* additions: the launch of the F-Factor app and F-Factor food line.

Throughout my years in private practice, clients would often ask me to recommend the highest fiber items available in the marketplace. I scoured the grocery aisle in search of cereals, bars, and snacks that fit F-Factor's guidelines. While I did find some products, there was much room for improvement— they could taste better, have more fiber, and be all-natural. There was a clear void in the marketplace for great-tasting high-fiber products and I knew if I could change that, it would enhance the F-Factor experience.

Today, I am pleased to announce the launch of the *new* F-Factor line of high-fiber products, which allows followers to get even more fiber in their diets—simply, deliciously, and naturally. The first products include bars and shakes. All are available on our website and from other online retailers now.

The F-Factor App will empower you to make better, more informed healthy-living decisions on the go. The F-Factor App is the only app to use F-Factor's proprietary conversion model for monitoring net carbs and fiber, allowing you to journal anytime, anywhere. In addition, the comprehensive tools keep track of your goals, weight loss, and body fat loss. When dining out or ordering in, the app provides you with #FFactorApproved options at your favorite restaurants so that you can eat-out/take-in with confidence. The F-Factor App is now available for download from the Apple App store and the Google Play store.

Together, the book, new products, and app will help you embark on your F-Factor journey. Congratulations on taking the first step to looking and feeling your very best!

**For more information and the latest updates, visit www.ffactor.com.**

All my best,

Tanya

# ACKNOWLEDGMENTS

THERE ARE many people I want to thank who contributed to my career in dietetics and the publication of this book.

First and foremost, thank you to my professors and counselors at New York University Department of Nutrition, Food Studies, and Public Health. It was at NYU that my passion for nutrition developed and thrived. Thank you to Marian Nestle, Ph.D., MPH, the Paulette Goddard Professor of Nutrition, Food Studies, and Public Health at NYU; Lisa Sasson, M.S., R.D., Clinical Assistant Professor; Carol Guber, M.S.; and Lisa Young, Ph.D., R.D., for your guidance and wisdom, and for inspiring me to pursue a career in dietetics.

Thank you to Dr. Ron Galluccio of East Side Medical and Cardiovascular Associates, P.C., and Dr. Jerome Zacks, Assistant Clinical Professor, Mount Sinai Medical Center. Thank you for believing in my abilities and for the countless patient referrals throughout the years. It was a privilege to work with you to help your patients to improve their health and quality of life. I am grateful for all the advice and wisdom that my agent, Fredi Friedman of Frederica S. Friedman & Company, Inc., has provided. I thank my editor, Marian Lizzi, for her endless support and enthusiasm. Her insights and editing skills have been invaluable in creating a book we can both be proud of.

This book would not be possible if it were not for the love and support of my family: my husband, Anthony Westreich, and our five children; my parents, Ken Zuckerbrot and Tamara Benson; and Leslie, Lenny, Ina, Andrew, and my beloved, late Grandma Claire. Thank you to my father, who taught me the value of education and supported me throughout my years of school and long into my career. Thank you to Leslie for spending hours reading my manuscript and helping me to organize my thoughts. Your editing skills are unparalleled. And to my amazing mother, who stayed late with me at my office on many evenings to analyze recipes and keep me company.

Thank you to the entire F-Factor family for working tirelessly in growing F-Factor into a company we can all be proud of: Gerry Casanova, Peter

Costello, Kristina Skordas, Jessica Robert, Jerzy Kurjanski, Aileen Cahill, Mark Weinrib, Shana Pantirer, R.D., Danielle Hamo, R.D., Maria Stavropoulos, R.D., Samantha Hass, R.D., Marleny Yac, Sean Kelley, and Tony Oddone.

Lastly, thank you to my clients, both past and present, for allowing me to share my love and knowledge of nutrition with you.

# CONTENTS

FOREWORD by Charles Stuart Platkin, J.D., MPH     xiii

**PART 1 ▪ A LOOK TO THE PAST, A LOOK TO THE FUTURE**

CHAPTER 1.   How Did We Get So Fat?
And Why the F-Factor Diet Is a Long-term Solution     3

**PART 2 ▪ WHY FIBER HOLDS THE KEY TO UNLOCKING WEIGHT LOSS FOR LIFE**

CHAPTER 2.   Your Quick Road Map: What You Need to Know
to Use the F-Factor Diet Successfully     23

CHAPTER 3.   Nutrition 101: The Food Groups     27

CHAPTER 4.   Do Carbohydrates Make You Fat? Dispelling the Myth     49

CHAPTER 5.   Fiber: The Secret Weapon for Healthy Weight Loss     59

**PART 3** ■ **THE PROGRAM: THE F-FACTOR DIET**

CHAPTER 6. Step 1: Jump-start Your Weight Loss 83

CHAPTER 7. Step 2: Continued Weight Loss 107

CHAPTER 8. Step 3: Maintenance—Eating for Life 135

CHAPTER 9. Dining Out and Ordering In 147

CHAPTER 10. Exercise to Empty Your Glycogen Stores 165

**PART 4** ■ **THE F-FACTOR DIET IN PRACTICE**

CHAPTER 11. The F-Factor Diet Recipes 177

APPENDIX A. Fiber Content of Popular Foods 265

APPENDIX B. Recommended Cereals and Breads 271

Index 275

About the Author 287

# FOREWORD

WHO WOULD have thought that your best bet for weight loss would be to eat *more* food—not less? That's exactly what Tanya Zuckerbrot suggests we do to get in shape. And it's all about eating more fiber. What is the big deal about fiber? Why devote an entire book to it?

As Tanya explains, fiber fills you up before it fills you out. Fiber-rich foods offer three major benefits to the weight-conscious person: they hold water in the stomach, they are digested slowly, and some of their calories are eliminated unabsorbed. High-fiber foods have a low caloric density (that is, you can eat a lot of them for a small amount of calories) because they are generally bulky and contain a lot of water. Fiber is the indigestible part of carbohydrates, so it really does satisfy you without contributing to weight gain. Keep in mind, it's the fiber *in the food* that's beneficial for weight loss; taking fiber pills isn't going to make you thin.

Fiber not only helps you lose weight but also is loaded with health benefits—it reduces your risk of heart disease and diabetes and helps lower cholesterol. Plus, fiber increases stool bulk, which can help prevent not only constipation but also hemorrhoids and possibly colon cancer.

The F-Factor Diet doesn't stop at just recommending fiber. F-Factor dieters will quickly discover the benefits of eating not only fiber but also protein, which makes you feel satisfied for a longer amount of time—without having to eat more. Foods high in protein slow the movement of food through the gastrointestinal tract; slower stomach emptying means you feel full longer and get hungrier later (increasing satiety), compared to diets that provide a lower protein content. Evidence from scientific studies also suggests high-protein meals lead to a reduced subsequent calorie intake. Also, eating foods that are low-fat, low-carb, and high in protein will help you to avoid other less healthy and high-calorie foods that do not keep you feeling full. And finally, research shows that the body uses more calories to digest protein than it does to burn fat or carbohydrates. The secret of the F-Factor Diet lies in combining high-fiber foods with lean protein at every meal.

The F-Factor Diet offers wonderful nutrition advice, with a number of intelligent twists, which all add up to a powerful weapon for those attempting to lose or control weight. Tanya Zuckerbrot has created a program that is as easy as any of the current trendy diets with two major differences: it's nutritionally sound, and it earns the approval of experts and dieters alike.

I've been working for years to educate the public about making the right choices when it comes to nutrition and health. With a plethora of diet books coming out every year, finally someone has come up with a sensible yet creative method to shed those unwanted pounds. I became a nutrition and public-health consumer advocate because I discovered firsthand how maddening and futile quick-weight-loss diets were—they were all simply a reduced-calorie diet plan disguised by some gimmick that limited the variety of foods I could eat. These prohibitive and overly strict diets have sparked hope in millions of dieters—only to fail them within months or even weeks. The F-Factor Diet provides dieters with the best of all worlds: the flexibility we all crave, the quick results of a fad diet, and the nutritional quality many of those diets lack.

A major downside of fad diets is ultimately regaining all the weight you may have lost—plus some additional weight. With all the talk about getting extra weight off your body, there's a lot less being said about how to keep it off—an elusive concept that is still poorly understood by the average dieter. Yet if you really think about it, weight maintenance is significantly more important and more difficult than losing weight. I can hear all of you saying,

"That's ridiculous. In order to keep weight off, you have to lose it first." That is certainly true, but think about how many times you've actually lost weight. Five, ten, maybe twenty times?

It is ironic that we focus on weight loss, when the real challenge is keeping weight off. Most popular diets work when it comes to losing weight, but few, if any, succeed when it comes to weight maintenance. Yet another reason why the F-Factor Diet can be so effective: the parameters of the diet allow enough flexibility so that you can maintain it forever, without feeling as though your food choices have been permanently limited.

Weight control is a forever process that requires dieters to make adjustments in their current behaviors—and that can be a difficult process, especially if they're trying to follow a rigid program. To be successful, your goal needs to be permanent weight loss, and one of the few ways to get there is by finding foods to eat—not finding foods *not* to eat. And that is what the F-Factor Diet provides—plenty of foods that you *can* eat. And those foods are highly nutritious and loaded with vitamins, minerals, and antioxidants.

Tanya Zuckerbrot gives you all the tools you need: a step-by-step program that incorporates easy-to-follow plans (including recipes) so you can map out the details of your personal long-term weight control program. You can finally lose the weight—without the struggle.

—*Charles Stuart Platkin,* PhD, J.D., MPH,
executive director, Hunter College,
New York City Food Policy Center;
distinguished lecturer, Hunter College,
City University of New York;
nationally syndicated health
columnist of "Diet Detective"

# A LOOK TO THE PAST, A LOOK TO THE FUTURE

# HOW DID WE GET SO FAT? AND WHY THE F-FACTOR DIET IS A LONG-TERM SOLUTION

*Thou shouldst eat to live; not live to eat.*
—SOCRATES (469 B.C.–399 B.C.)

YOU NOTICE it at the beach.

You observe it in the fans at sporting events.

A quick look around the mall and there is no denying it: Americans are fatter than ever.

Currently, 70 percent of American adults are overweight, and half of them are obese. Yet merely three decades ago, less than 50 percent of the American population was overweight. As the years passed, somehow our waistlines kept expanding. It wouldn't be such a big deal if the problem were simply aesthetic. But excess weight correlates with increased risk of heart disease, high blood pressure, stroke, diabetes, infertility, gallbladder disease, osteoarthritis, and many forms of cancer. The *Journal of the American Medical Association* reported in 2004 that being overweight could soon overtake tobacco as the leading cause of preventable death in the United States. We clearly have reason to worry.

A recent survey published in the National Institute of Public Health publication reports that, in the United States on any given day, 44 percent of men and almost 66 percent of women are trying to lose weight. Last year alone, Americans spent billions of dollars on weight-loss products, health club memberships, diet foods, liposuctions, and gastric bypass operations.[1] And where did investments in these supposed panaceas get us? Despite our attempts to lose weight, this country's population is currently the heaviest it has ever been. Our individual weight problems have become a national crisis.

After low-fat diets failed to put an end to the epidemic of obesity, low-carb diets appeared to be the solution to Americans' struggle with weight. We tried diets like Atkins and South Beach, and in doing so, cut out bread, fruit, milk, yogurt, and even vegetables in order to whittle down our waistlines. But after a decade of low-carb eating, the truth remains: Americans are fatter than ever.

The problem with low-carb diets is the same as with low-fat diets, and with the numerous other failed diets of the past: their focus is on *eliminating* foods in order to lose weight. Whether you are cutting out fat or carbohydrates, the result is that you end up craving the foods that have become taboo. Who wants to feel deprived of their favorite foods in order to maintain a

> A recent survey published in the National Institute of Public Health publication reports that, in the United States on any given day, 44 percent of men and almost 66 percent of women are trying to lose weight.

> In 2015, according to the United States Centers for Disease Control and Prevention, over 70 percent of American adults are overweight, whereas three decades ago the incidence of overweight adults was well under 50 percent.

1. M. Lemonick, "How We Grew So Big," *Time* 163, no. 23 (June 7, 2004).

desired weight? A life without bagels for breakfast, pasta at Italian restaurants, or rice with your Chinese food? That's crazy! And that is also why most diets are temporary.

## How Did We Get So Fat?

The advent and growth of industrialization, jumbo portion sizes, and fad diets produced a predictable, understandable, and inevitable consequence—an epidemic of obesity and diet-related diseases.

### Industrialization

You might equate industrialization with advancements in engineering, economy, and human resources. While sounding promising, industrialization applied to food processing has negatively affected Americans' nutrition.

Before industrialization, whole grains were left whole. Breads and rice were brown; fruits and vegetables were eaten just the way they came out of the ground or off the tree. These foods were nutritious, rich in vitamins, and full of fiber. Now, however, our supermarkets stock white bread, sweetened fruit drinks, and instant mashed potatoes—the legacy of agricultural industrialization that has left us in a fiber deficit.

The absence of fiber in Americans' diets is a major risk factor for weight gain. Despite the American Dietetic Association recommending that Americans eat 25 to 38 grams of fiber per day, the average American currently eats only 15 grams of fiber a day. Not eating enough fiber leads people to feel hungry and to overeat throughout the day.

Snacking contributes to one-fourth of Americans' daily caloric intake. And when we snack, what do we choose? Chips, cookies, crackers, sweetened beverages, and frozen desserts, all of which contain virtually no fiber. People who eat these foods to try to satisfy their appetites only find themselves hun-

> Despite the American Dietetic Association recommending that Americans eat 25 to 38 grams of fiber per day, the average American currently eats only 15 grams of fiber a day.

gry again soon after. Diets based on such refined foods create a vicious cycle of eating and hunger all day long.

To add insult to injury, refined foods are available everywhere, all of the time. Walk down the cookie or snack-chip aisles in your supermarket, and you find hundreds of choices. Delis, food courts, and vending machines present the opportunity to snack around the clock. Gas stations used to sell only gas—now they have been remodeled to house a food market inside. Going to the gas station no longer means just filling up your tank; it now is an opportunity to fill up your belly. An increase in convenience has provoked a shift to frequent "grazing"—eating small but cumulatively hefty snacks, as opposed to regular meals.

As technological advances have made food ever more varied, convenient, and tasty, the feeble willpower of the American public has been unable to cope. Most people know the rule of thermodynamics: calories in versus calories out. If you eat more calories than you burn, you will gain weight. Americans are not only eating more (the average American consumes 2,640 calories a day, up from 1,970 calories in 1978), we are also moving less.

Technology has not only made food more varied and convenient, it has almost completely removed natural physical exercise from most Americans' day-to-day lives. In the early nineteenth century, if you wanted ice cream, you would have to walk out to the pasture, milk the cow, carry the milk back to the farmhouse, mix in sugar and eggs, add salt to the ice, and churn the whole thing for hours until it froze. A person would burn a few hundred calories in the process. Now if people crave ice cream, they only have to walk to the refrigerator or drive to the nearest convenience store for a pint of Ben & Jerry's.

Cars, washing machines, elevators, escalators, and moving sidewalks at the airport have reduced physical exertion. Watching television for hours, sitting

> Americans are not only eating more (the average American consumes 2,640 calories a day, up from 1,970 calories in 1978), we are also moving less.

in front of a computer, and playing video games create the perfect recipe for weight gain.

Eating refined foods frequently and moving less are not the only problems. Ever-expanding food portions are also to blame.

## Out-of-Control Portion Sizes

Advances in agriculture and farming followed industrialization. Never has food in this country been so abundant. This country produces 3,800 calories of food for every man, woman, and child every day—almost twice as many as most people need.[2] The surplus of food translates into whopping portions at low prices, and Americans are eating them up. Larger portions seem to make consumers feel that they are getting their money's worth. And the food companies are responding.

With the exception of sliced white bread, the sizes of sodas, hamburgers, French fries, pizza slices, and other foods commonly available for immediate consumption exceed standard portions determined by the U.S. Department of Agriculture (USDA) and the Food and Drug Administration (FDA). Cookies, cooked pastas, muffins, steaks, and bagels exceeded USDA standards by 700 percent, 480 percent, 333 percent, 224 percent, and 195 percent respectively.[3]

In the 1950s, McDonald's offered one size, a 2-ounce portion of French fries that contained 200 calories. Starting in 2004, the 2-ounce size was offered only on the kids' menu, and adults were offered a 7-ounce French fry serving with 610 calories. In 1997, Starbucks took the 8-ounce Short, its smallest size, off the menu when it introduced the 20-ounce Venti (the Extra Large). Now the 12-ounce Tall is the smallest choice. Larger portions are attractive to customers because the relative prices discourage the choice of smaller portions.[4] How many times at the concession stand at the movies have you heard the vendor tell you that for a few cents more, you can get the next size up? Unfortunately, you are not just getting more value for your money; you are also getting more calories. A Coke and buttered popcorn combination has 688 calories, while a value pack (large Coke and buttered popcorn) has

2. L. Lindner, "Fat of the Land," *Eating Well*, 2001, 15–21.
3. L. R. Young and M. Nestle, "The Contribution of Expanding Portion Sizes to the U.S. Obesity Epidemic." *American Journal of Public Health* 92 (2002): 246–49.
4. M. Nestle, *Food Politics: How the Food Industry Influences Nutrition and Health* (Berkeley: University of California Press, 2003).

2,174 calories (based on small popcorn serving size 5 cups; large popcorn serving size 20 cups; small Coke serving size 18 oz, large Coke serving size 44 oz).

Bigger portions are everywhere. At fast-food joints and convenience stores, the trend is hard to miss—7-Eleven offers the 48-ounce Double Gulp, and the muffins at Au Bon Pain are the size of softballs. Not only have food portions increased but, according to the National Restaurant Association in Washington, D.C., our plates have grown, too. The 10-inch plate was once the industry standard; now 12-inch plates are the norm. Servings are so big that in some restaurants you get two or three times more than you need. A typical meal at an ordinary restaurant contains 1,200 calories, and that's without the dessert or appetizer.

More calories equal more weight gain, pure and simple.

Larger restaurant portions have become an increased problem because Americans eat out more frequently than they used to. Twenty years ago, most people ate in restaurants only on special occasions. Today, the typical American eats out 4.5 times a week.[5]

Larger portions have even entered our homes. Serving sizes in popular cookbooks, such as *The Joy of Cooking,* are getting "hearty" as well. In 1960, a brownie recipe in *The Joy of Cooking* yielded 30 brownies. Today, in its most current edition, the brownie recipe calls for exactly the same proportions as the original, but instead of the original 30-brownie yield, the recipe now yields only 16 brownies. That means each brownie is almost twice as big, with double the amount of calories as the original.[6]

Even "diet" foods, including certain brands of frozen dinners, now come in larger sizes. For instance, in 1996, Stouffer's introduced a packaged food

> In the 1950s, McDonald's offered one size, a 2-ounce portion of French fries that contained 200 calories. Starting in 2004, the 2-ounce size was offered only on the kids' menu, and adults were offered a 7-ounce French fry serving with 610 calories.

5. Zagat, "The State of American Dining in 2016" (January 26, 2016).
6. L. R. Young and M. Nestle, "The Contribution of Expanding Portion Sizes to the U.S. Obesity Epidemic," *American Journal of Public Health* 92 (2002): 246–49.

line called Lean Cuisine Hearty Portions that weighed 50 percent more than the original, and which of course had more calories.[7]

The result of these larger portions is that Americans' conception of a serving has become skewed. Standard portion sizes recommended by the American Dietetic Association have become a thing of the past. Now when we are served a standard portion, it seems measly.

> The official Nutrition Facts serving size for spaghetti and tomato sauce is 1 cup, with 250 calories and 5 grams of fat. A typical restaurant serves 3.5 cups of pasta and sauce, weighing in at over 850 calories and 17 grams of fat.

## Fad Diets

The greater the prevalence of obesity, the more alluring is the latest fad diet promising fast and easy weight loss. American dieters' eagerness to find the magic weight-loss bullet has led them from no-fat diets to high-protein diets. The problem now is that many Americans no longer know what they should be eating.

In 1981, Americans were introduced to *Dr. Atkins' Diet Revolution* (Bantam). The diet was high-protein and high-fat with minimal carbohydrates. People lost weight but found a diet without carbohydrates difficult to maintain. In the late 1980s, studies from the American Heart Association reported that dietary fat increased the risk factors for cardiovascular disease. Americans took this information to heart, banished fat from their diets, and entered the fat-free decade of the 1990s. The 1990s introduced Americans to fat-free cookies, cakes, chips, and every food imaginable that could be remade without fat.

Americans loved the concept of fat-free foods because, unlike other diets that made you count calories, eating fat-free meant no calorie watching. If a

7. *Tufts University Health & Nutrition Letter* 20, no. 4 (June 2002).

food was fat-free, that was the green light to dig in! Americans began eating large bagels (no cream cheese), bowls of pasta (no cream or oil, just tomato sauce) and large quantities of fat-free pastries from companies like SnackWell's and Entenmann's.

For breakfast, instead of two eggs and a piece of buttered toast (265 calories, 15 grams fat), a fat-free dieter opted for a 1,000-calorie fat-free muffin. And for a snack, instead of eating two 100-calorie Oreo cookies with 5 grams of fat, people would eat half a box of SnackWell's cookies, which contained 400 calories, and no fat. Although they were eating more calories, people assumed that, since there was no fat, they could get away with it. Wow, were they fooled!

Unfortunately, fat-free dieting led to more weight gain. By 1990, Americans were 6 percent heavier than a decade earlier.[8] Calories appeared to be a major culprit. Despite the drop in fat intake, average calorie intake increased from 1,970 calories a day in 1978 to 2,200 in 1990.[9]

Most fat-free product manufacturers replaced the fat in the recipes with sugar and starch. Many fat-free foods ended up with the same number of or even more calories than the full-fat original. And the biggest problem with eating fat-free foods is that a person never actually feels full or satisfied. That is because fat adds satiety to a meal. Without a little fat, you feel hungry soon after you finish eating. So people ate more, and eventually gained more weight. Once again, weight-conscious Americans were let down by another diet trend.

Trends come full circle. In response to the failure of fat-free diets, we returned to the high-fat, high-protein diets of the 1970s. The Atkins diet made a comeback, and low-carb foods quickly replaced all those now-condemned low-fat products on the supermarket shelves. We threw out the offending SnackWell's and replaced them with Atkins bars and Carb Smart ice cream. The late 1990s were spent eating steak, butter, bacon, and eggs. As long as there were no carbohydrates in a food, it was okay to eat it. Nevertheless, by the end of the '90s, despite cutting out carbohydrates, 64.5 percent of Americans were overweight, up from 44.8 percent in 1960.[10]

8. M. Flynn, M.S., R.D., "Fat-Free Foods: Diet Aid or Dieter's Downfall?" *Environmental Nutrition* 18 (April 1995): 6.
9. Ibid.
10. National Center for Health Statistics, *Health, United States, 2002* (Hyattsville, MD: 2002).

The essential problem with diets is that people don't stay on them very long. The average weight-loss attempt is four weeks for women, six for men.[11] So until you pick a way of eating that's going to last all your life, you haven't found the "right" diet.

How many of you have gone on a very low calorie diet for, say, two weeks and lost 5 to 10 pounds? Whether you chose the Scarsdale diet, the grapefruit diet, the cabbage soup diet, Slimfast, or Atkins, eventually you were bound to be disappointed. That's because diets are a temporary solution to a lifelong problem.

When people reach their weight loss goal, many go off their diet. The first thing they end up eating are the foods they felt most deprived of. If they were on Atkins, they might go for a bowl of pasta or a bagel with cream cheese. If they were on a low-fat diet, they dive into high-fat items like steak and French fries.

Returning to our old eating habits invites the weight to come back. Once the weight returns, you find yourself on a diet again a few weeks later. It is a vicious cycle:

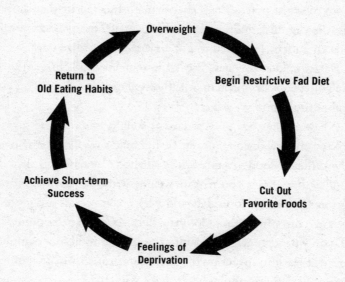

11. A. Spake, "The Science of Slimming," *U.S. News & World Report* (June 16, 2003): 34–40.

## The Ultimate Solution: Why the F-Factor Diet Is Different

The good news is that we finally have a permanent solution.

The F-Factor Diet is the last diet you will ever need. Now for the first time when you begin a diet, you won't be focusing on which foods you must *omit*. Instead you will consider the foods you need to *add* to your diet in order to lose weight and keep it off. And those foods are probably just the ones you've been so carefully avoiding these past few years—carbohydrates.

Yes, you read correctly. On the F-Factor Diet, you *must* eat carbohydrates in order to start dropping pounds.

So what is the F factor?

*Fiber!*

Fiber may not be the sexy answer you were hoping for, but when it comes to losing weight and improving your health, nothing works better.

## How the F-Factor Diet Began

During my years of practice as a dietitian, I observed firsthand the feelings of deprivation, reward, guilt, and lowered self-esteem my clients have experienced on other diets. I decided to put an end to diet misery.

The F-Factor Diet is a new way of looking at food. Instead of focusing on cutting out foods like protein or carbohydrates, one focuses on *adding* the *right* kind of foods into your diet.

The F-Factor Diet not only promotes weight loss but also gives you the tools to keep the weight off forever. In the first few chapters, you will learn about the different food groups, how your body metabolizes them, and my magic bullet that allows you to lose weight without starving yourself. This information equips you to understand why certain foods are more likely to cause weight gain, while other foods can help you shed extra pounds. Within no time, you will reprogram your mind to look at food in a completely new way. You will learn to dispel myths like "lean proteins include only chicken and fish, not beef" or "carbohydrates make you fat."

Unlike most diets, you never go off the F-Factor diet. Once you reach your weight-loss goal, you enter a maintenance phase that enables you to keep the weight off effortlessly. By the time you reach the maintenance phase, you will have established a healthy, well-balanced lifestyle with no taboo foods. Even the most decadent foods can be eaten in moderation. You will have broken the vicious cycle of fad dieting and bad eating habits forever.

## How Does the Diet Work?

The success of the F-Factor Diet lies in combining high-fiber foods with lean protein at every meal.

Why fiber? Fiber is the indigestible component of carbohydrates that provides bulk *without any calories*. Fiber fills you up without filling you out and helps to eliminate hunger pangs associated with dieting. Fiber speeds up weight loss, pure and simple. And the best part is, you get to eat carbohydrates from day one of the F-Factor Diet. After years of avoiding the bread basket, the F-Factor Diet brings carbohydrates back to your table.

The F-Factor Diet is about more than just adding fiber to your diet. You must eat protein, too.

From the first day, you can choose from foods like chicken, steak, eggs, turkey, veal, lamb, fish, shrimp, scallops, and even lobster. Clinical evidence shows that fiber and protein have a high satiety benefit in calorie-controlled diets and in weight reduction. The combination of fiber and protein keeps you feeling full for the longest period of time on the fewest calories. The fuller you feel after a meal, the less likely you'll be to overeat at the next meal; and, therefore, the more likely you'll be to lose weight.

By concentrating on what you should be *adding* to your diet instead of what you're cutting out, you will always feel full and satisfied. In essence,

Fiber and protein at every meal
Makes losing weight no big deal.

Once you begin the program, you'll understand the power of these words to help you lose weight and keep it off for good.

It isn't hard to see why high-fiber diets haven't been popular in the past. When most people think of fiber, images of grainy fiber supplements, dry bran, and prunes come to mind. Perhaps that is why most Americans don't come close to eating the recommended 35–38 grams of fiber a day. Typically, the average American gets only 9 to 15 grams of fiber a day. The very fact that Americans spend $1.3 billion on laxatives is a clear indication that we do not get the fiber we need.

On the F-Factor Diet, you don't have to suffer with "good-for-you" fiber foods to get fiber into your diet. For example, you can choose a juicy pear. A medium pear has 6 grams of fiber compared to 3.9 grams in a serving of dried prunes. That's 35 percent more fiber! Pears aren't the only tasty food packed with fiber. Blueberries, almonds, cereal, crackers, soups, salads, whole-wheat bread and pasta are among the delicious foods you will be eating on the F-Factor Diet.

While following the F-Factor Diet, you will not only experience weight loss but also better health. You will see improvements in the condition of your hair and the clarity of your complexion, and you will feel more energetic, healthy, and satisfied.

Following this diet will also mean that you will improve your cholesterol levels and reduce your risk of cardiovascular disease, adult-onset diabetes, and even cancer. High-fiber carbohydrates are filled with powerful antioxidants and phytochemicals, which prevent disease and premature aging.

## Three Steps Make the Diet Easy As 1-2-3

From day one on the F-Factor Diet you will be putting the carbohydrates that you've banished from your plate back into your diet. You will be eating three servings of high-fiber carbohydrates per day, including cereal, fruit, and crackers. And you can eat a variety of lean protein and all the vegetables you want.

After approximately two weeks on Step 1 of the F-Factor Diet, you are guaranteed to have lost between 4 and 6 pounds. You will then begin Step 2, at which point you will be adding 3 more servings of high-fiber carbohydrates, such as bread, rice, and even pasta. You can expect to lose 2 pounds every week on Step 2, until you reach your weight-loss goal.

Once you have arrived successfully at your desired weight, you enter Step 3, the maintenance phase, where you will be eating a total of 9 servings of carbohydrates a day, every day, for the rest of your life. No food, even the most decadent, will be forbidden as long as it is eaten in moderation. You will have reduced your risk for heart disease, diabetes, and cancer while shedding pounds, boosting your energy levels, and taking control of your health and happiness.

## Why the F-Factor Diet Is Different

If all this sounds too good to be true, I assure you that it isn't. In fact, it's those other diets you've probably been on and off all your life that make unrealistic promises. After all, if they hadn't failed to live up to their promises, you wouldn't be reading this book.

So why should you believe the F-Factor Diet will be any different? Because none of those other diets was created by anyone with a background of education in nutrition. Dr. Atkins (*Atkins for Life*), Dr. Agatston (the South Beach Diet), and Dr. Sears (the Zone Diet) may all be successful cardiologists, but none of them is a dietitian.

It is a known fact that doctors do not study nutrition intensively and most are required only to take one or two nutrition courses during their medical education. Therefore, when it comes to offering dietetic advice, most doctors can proffer the basics, but when it comes to giving specific detailed counseling, doctors often refer their patients to a registered dietitian. Doctors are busy seeing patients throughout the day and don't have the time to create menus. Referring patients to a registered dietitian not only saves them valuable time but also ensures that their patients receive the best nutritional care possible.

# Why You Need a Dietitian's Experience

I am not only a board-certified dietitian, I also hold a master's degree in nutrition and food studies from New York University and have completed a dietetic residency at New York University Hospital. My practice began with doctor referrals, primarily cardiologists and endocrinologists, who sent patients to me to lower cholesterol and control diabetes.

I created programs for both these patient populations to help them improve their clinical conditions. A common thread among the diets I created for these two groups of patients was a high fiber content. (Fiber helps to lower cholesterol by binding with it and pulling it out of one's system, and it is crucial for diabetics because it slows down the digestion of carbohydrates, therefore avoiding a sharp increase in blood sugar levels.)

All patients not only saw improvements in their clinical conditions but all also lost weight! Patients felt full, satisfied, and had improved energy throughout the day. It was then that I realized that fiber has the amazing ability to help with weight loss. I adopted this principle and created the F-Factor Diet.

Over the past two decades, I have helped tens of thousands of patients to lose weight and to improve their health. My practical hands-on experience teaches me what works for patients and what doesn't. I have spent hours talking with patients about obstacles that occur while dieting and what motivates them to stick to a program. I have been able to use this patient information to create a program that tastes delicious, is easy to follow, and guarantees weight loss.

What I found is that people want a simple diet, one that allows them to dine out without difficulty, that tastes good and leaves them feeling satisfied, one that improves their health and enables them to lose weight without feelings of deprivation or denial. The result is the F-Factor Diet.

I named this program the F-Factor Diet because "fiber" is the dirty little word no one wants to hear. When people think of fiber they may think of roughage, bloating, and dry, tasteless food. Not an inviting image. Yet fiber is actually found in many delicious foods that you will enjoy adding to your diet. For me, and for my patients, fiber is the secret to losing weight and keeping it off.

*A review of published studies shows that people on a diet that is both low in fat and high in fiber lose three times as much weight as people on a low-fat diet alone.* My patients experienced the same result.[12] Fiber makes you feel full, so you eat less. Also, foods that are high in fiber—such as beans, fruits, vegetables, and whole grains—tend to be low in calories, so you can consume a greater volume of food. Think about how much more satisfying it is to eat an apple

---

12. M. Yao and S. B. Roberts, "Dietary Energy Density and Weight Regulation," *Nutrition Review* 59, no. 5 (August 2001): 129–39, and W. J. Pasman, W. H. Saris, M. A. Wauters, et al., "Effect of One Week of Fibre Supplementation on Hunger and Satiety Ratings and Energy Intake," *Appetite* 29, no. 1 (August 1997): 77–87.

(3 grams of fiber; 80 calories) than to drink an 8-ounce glass of apple juice (no fiber; 110 calories).

## Proof of Real Results

For over twenty years, I have been using this diet plan with hundreds of my patients, including high-powered executives, Radio City Rockettes, real-estate developers, film producers, models, actors, diplomats, flight attendants, policemen, and stay-at-home moms.

On the F-Factor Diet, many of my clients lowered their cholesterol so much that they were able to discontinue cholesterol-lowering medication entirely and greatly reduce their risk for cardiovascular disease. Those clients with type 2 diabetes have been able to control their insulin levels through diet alone. They all reported new levels of energy. They all have lost weight almost effortlessly, and most importantly, have kept it off.

Food fads come and go, but the F-Factor Diet is based on a dietitian's understanding of anatomy and physiology. This diet's scientific principles don't change with the diet tides. Once you understand how your body digests, uti-

---

The terms *overweight* and *obese* are defined by a Body Mass Index (BMI), a direct calculation based on an individual's height and weight. BMI generally relates to body fat. As BMI increases, especially from values equal to or greater than 30, so does a person's health risk. Being overweight (a BMI of 25 to 30) or being obese (a BMI greater than 30) increases the risk of having high blood pressure, heart disease, stroke, diabetes, certain types of cancer, arthritis, and breathing problems.[13]

To find out your BMI, check the chart on page 19. (BMI is not gender specific.)

For example, a 5'6" (66 inches tall) woman who weighs 126 pounds has a BMI of 20, which falls in the "healthy weight" category. Yet a woman of the same height (5'6") who weighs 174 pounds would fall into the "overweight" category.

---

13. M. C. Hochber, M. Lethbridge-Cejku, W. W. Scott Jr., et al., "The Association of Body Weight, Body Fatness, and Body Fat Distribution with Osteoarthritis of the Knee: Data from the Baltimore Longitudinal Study of Aging," *Journal of Rheumatology* 22 (1995): 488–93.

lizes, and stores carbohydrates in Chapter 4, you will understand why certain foods are more likely than others to cause weight gain. You will see that the only way carbohydrates can make you fat is if you eat more of them than your body can use. With that new understanding, you, too, will embrace the principles of the F-Factor Diet and make them a way of life. You will be eating carbohydrates and losing weight without any sense of deprivation—and you will look and feel better than ever before.

# Body Mass Index Table

| BMI | 19 | 20 | 21 | 22 | 23 | 24 | 25 | 26 | 27 | 28 | 29 | 30 | 31 | 32 | 33 | 34 | 35 | 36 | 37 | 38 | 39 | 40 | 41 | 42 | 43 | 44 | 45 | 46 | 47 | 48 | 49 | 50 | 51 | 52 | 53 | 54 |
|---|---|---|---|---|---|---|---|---|---|---|---|---|---|---|---|---|---|---|---|---|---|---|---|---|---|---|---|---|---|---|---|---|---|---|---|---|
| **Category** | Normal | | | | | | Overweight | | | | | Obese | | | | | | | | | | Extreme Obesity | | | | | | | | | | | | | | | |
| **Height (inches)** | Body Weight (pounds) | | | | | | | | | | | | | | | | | | | | | | | | | | | | | | | | | | | | |
| 58 | 91 | 96 | 100 | 105 | 110 | 115 | 119 | 124 | 129 | 134 | 138 | 143 | 148 | 153 | 158 | 162 | 167 | 172 | 177 | 181 | 186 | 191 | 196 | 201 | 205 | 210 | 215 | 220 | 224 | 229 | 234 | 239 | 244 | 248 | 253 | 258 |
| 59 | 94 | 99 | 104 | 109 | 114 | 119 | 124 | 128 | 133 | 138 | 143 | 148 | 153 | 158 | 163 | 168 | 173 | 178 | 183 | 188 | 193 | 198 | 203 | 208 | 212 | 217 | 222 | 227 | 232 | 237 | 242 | 247 | 252 | 257 | 262 | 267 |
| 60 | 97 | 102 | 107 | 112 | 118 | 123 | 128 | 133 | 138 | 143 | 148 | 153 | 158 | 163 | 168 | 174 | 179 | 184 | 189 | 194 | 199 | 204 | 209 | 215 | 220 | 225 | 230 | 235 | 240 | 245 | 250 | 255 | 261 | 266 | 271 | 276 |
| 61 | 100 | 106 | 111 | 116 | 122 | 127 | 132 | 137 | 143 | 148 | 153 | 158 | 164 | 169 | 174 | 180 | 185 | 190 | 195 | 201 | 206 | 211 | 217 | 222 | 227 | 232 | 238 | 243 | 248 | 254 | 259 | 264 | 269 | 275 | 280 | 285 |
| 62 | 104 | 109 | 115 | 120 | 126 | 131 | 136 | 142 | 147 | 153 | 158 | 164 | 169 | 175 | 180 | 186 | 191 | 196 | 202 | 207 | 213 | 218 | 224 | 229 | 235 | 240 | 246 | 251 | 256 | 262 | 267 | 273 | 278 | 284 | 289 | 295 |
| 63 | 107 | 113 | 118 | 124 | 130 | 135 | 141 | 146 | 152 | 158 | 163 | 169 | 175 | 180 | 186 | 191 | 197 | 203 | 208 | 214 | 220 | 225 | 231 | 237 | 242 | 248 | 254 | 259 | 265 | 270 | 278 | 282 | 287 | 293 | 299 | 304 |
| 64 | 110 | 116 | 122 | 128 | 134 | 140 | 145 | 151 | 157 | 163 | 169 | 174 | 180 | 186 | 192 | 197 | 204 | 209 | 215 | 221 | 227 | 232 | 238 | 244 | 250 | 256 | 262 | 267 | 273 | 279 | 285 | 291 | 296 | 302 | 308 | 314 |
| 65 | 114 | 120 | 126 | 132 | 138 | 144 | 150 | 156 | 162 | 168 | 174 | 180 | 186 | 192 | 198 | 204 | 210 | 216 | 222 | 228 | 234 | 240 | 246 | 252 | 258 | 264 | 270 | 276 | 282 | 288 | 294 | 300 | 306 | 312 | 318 | 324 |
| 66 | 118 | 124 | 130 | 136 | 142 | 148 | 155 | 161 | 167 | 173 | 178 | 186 | 192 | 198 | 204 | 210 | 216 | 223 | 229 | 235 | 241 | 247 | 253 | 260 | 266 | 272 | 278 | 284 | 291 | 297 | 303 | 309 | 315 | 322 | 328 | 334 |
| 67 | 121 | 127 | 134 | 140 | 146 | 153 | 159 | 166 | 172 | 178 | 185 | 191 | 198 | 204 | 211 | 217 | 223 | 230 | 236 | 242 | 249 | 255 | 261 | 268 | 274 | 280 | 287 | 293 | 299 | 306 | 312 | 319 | 325 | 331 | 338 | 344 |
| 68 | 125 | 131 | 138 | 144 | 151 | 158 | 164 | 171 | 177 | 184 | 190 | 197 | 203 | 210 | 216 | 223 | 230 | 236 | 243 | 249 | 256 | 262 | 269 | 276 | 282 | 289 | 295 | 302 | 308 | 315 | 322 | 328 | 335 | 341 | 348 | 354 |
| 69 | 128 | 135 | 142 | 149 | 155 | 162 | 169 | 176 | 182 | 189 | 196 | 203 | 209 | 216 | 223 | 230 | 236 | 243 | 250 | 257 | 263 | 270 | 277 | 284 | 291 | 297 | 304 | 311 | 318 | 324 | 331 | 338 | 345 | 351 | 358 | 365 |
| 70 | 132 | 139 | 146 | 153 | 160 | 167 | 174 | 181 | 188 | 195 | 202 | 209 | 216 | 222 | 229 | 236 | 243 | 250 | 257 | 264 | 271 | 278 | 285 | 292 | 299 | 306 | 313 | 320 | 327 | 334 | 341 | 348 | 355 | 362 | 369 | 376 |
| 71 | 136 | 143 | 150 | 157 | 165 | 172 | 179 | 186 | 193 | 200 | 208 | 215 | 222 | 229 | 236 | 243 | 250 | 257 | 265 | 272 | 279 | 286 | 293 | 301 | 308 | 315 | 322 | 329 | 338 | 343 | 351 | 358 | 365 | 372 | 379 | 386 |
| 72 | 140 | 147 | 154 | 162 | 169 | 177 | 184 | 191 | 199 | 206 | 213 | 221 | 228 | 235 | 242 | 250 | 258 | 265 | 272 | 279 | 287 | 294 | 302 | 309 | 316 | 324 | 331 | 338 | 346 | 353 | 361 | 368 | 375 | 383 | 390 | 397 |
| 73 | 144 | 151 | 159 | 166 | 174 | 182 | 189 | 197 | 204 | 212 | 219 | 227 | 235 | 242 | 250 | 257 | 265 | 272 | 280 | 288 | 295 | 302 | 310 | 318 | 325 | 333 | 340 | 348 | 355 | 363 | 371 | 378 | 386 | 393 | 401 | 408 |
| 74 | 148 | 155 | 163 | 171 | 179 | 186 | 194 | 202 | 210 | 218 | 225 | 233 | 241 | 249 | 256 | 264 | 272 | 280 | 287 | 295 | 303 | 311 | 319 | 326 | 334 | 342 | 350 | 358 | 365 | 373 | 381 | 389 | 396 | 404 | 412 | 420 |
| 75 | 152 | 160 | 168 | 176 | 184 | 192 | 299 | 208 | 216 | 224 | 232 | 240 | 248 | 256 | 264 | 272 | 279 | 287 | 295 | 303 | 311 | 319 | 327 | 335 | 343 | 351 | 359 | 367 | 375 | 383 | 391 | 399 | 407 | 415 | 423 | 431 |
| 76 | 156 | 164 | 172 | 180 | 189 | 197 | 205 | 213 | 221 | 230 | 238 | 246 | 254 | 263 | 271 | 279 | 287 | 295 | 304 | 312 | 320 | 328 | 336 | 344 | 353 | 361 | 369 | 377 | 385 | 394 | 402 | 410 | 418 | 426 | 435 | 443 |

Source: Evidence Report of Clinical Guidelines on the Identification, Evaluation, and Treatment of Overweight and Obesity in Adults, 1998. NIH/National Heart, Lung, and Blood Institute (NHLBI).

# WHY FIBER HOLDS THE KEY TO UNLOCKING WEIGHT LOSS FOR LIFE

YOUR QUICK ROAD MAP:
WHAT YOU NEED TO KNOW TO
USE THE F-FACTOR DIET SUCCESSFULLY

CONGRATULATIONS ON deciding to explore the F-Factor Diet. By doing so, you have begun a journey not just to lose weight but also to enhance your health and probability for longevity. With so much to benefit, it is understandable that you are excited to begin the F-Factor Diet.

Before you can start this program, you will need some basic information about why and how the F-Factor Diet works. One thing I guarantee is that after beginning this program, you will never look at food in the same way. You will still love to eat, but you will do so with an appreciation and understanding you may not have possessed before.

No more deprivation. No more diet gimmicks. The F-Factor Diet is about learning, finally, how to eat a well-balanced diet for life.

## A Quick Road Map

- Chapter 3 teaches you about the different food groups and defines which are carbohydrates and which are not. This knowledge provides the building blocks for the F-Factor Diet to work.

- Chapter 4 describes how your body digests and uses carbohydrates for fuel. By the end of Chapter 4, you will embrace the fact that eating carbohydrates does not lead to weight gain. The next step is to learn about which carbohydrates are best for you.
- Chapter 5 introduces fiber, the indigestible portion of carbohydrates. You will learn about the health benefits of fiber and how adding fiber-rich foods to your diet will enable you to lose unwanted pounds without feeling hungry or deprived.

With the education you received in Chapters 3, 4, and 5 under your belt, you are ready to begin the F-Factor Diet.

## Why Not Start with Chapter 6?

You may be tempted to jump right to Chapter 6 to begin this diet, but skipping Chapters 3, 4, and 5 won't help you to lose weight any faster. In fact, without comprehending the information in those chapters, you will have a difficult time following the diet.

So take a few extra minutes to read through Chapters 3, 4, and 5, and I assure you this reading-time investment will pay off in the long run!

### Test Your "FIQ" (Fiber Knowledge)

How much do you really know about fiber? A recent study conducted by the National Fiber Council revealed that most Americans lack basic information about dietary fiber and the important role it can play in the prevention of many prevalent health conditions. Test your knowledge with a few of the survey questions asked. Later in the book you'll find all the information you need to boost your fiber for lasting health and weight loss.

1. On average, how much fiber should Americans be eating on a daily basis?
   a. 5–15 grams
   b. 16–25 grams
   c. 26–38 grams
   d. 39–50 grams

2. Which of the following health benefits *cannot* be linked to a high-fiber diet?

   a. Helps prevent heart disease

   b. Helps improve vision

   c. Helps lower blood cholesterol

   d. Helps manage diabetes

   e. Helps manage weight

3. Which of the following foods *does not* contain a significant amount of fiber?

   a. Raspberries

   b. Steak

   c. Whole-grain breads

   d. Bananas

   e. Nuts

   f. Broccoli

   g. They all contain a significant amount of fiber

   h. None of the above

4. How many medium-sized apples would you need to eat to get the recommended amount of fiber you need in one day?

   a. 2

   b. 4

   c. 6

   d. 8

   e. None of the above

5. What age groups would benefit from the health benefits of daily fiber intake?

   a. 12–25

   b. 26–40

   c. 41–60

   d. 61–80

   e. All of the above

Answers:  1. c   2. b   3. b   4. d   5. e

# NUTRITION 101:
# THE FOOD GROUPS

*Give a man a fish and you feed him for a day.*
*Teach him to fish and you feed him for a lifetime.*
——LAO TZU

LAO TZU'S message resonates throughout life's experiences, and never more so than during the attempt to diet. For most people, maintaining a healthy weight is a lifelong struggle.

If you simply give people a diet without teaching *why* it works, you have offered a short-term solution to a lifelong problem. Some people may follow the diet for a limited time, but unless they comprehend the program's principles, it is unlikely many of them will stay with it. Think about it—you are much more likely to follow rules when you understand why they exist.

In my years of counseling patients, I found that those who comprehended the principles of the F-Factor Diet exhibited the greatest compliance to the program and therefore achieved the greatest weight loss. Learning *why* you should eat certain foods and *how* those foods cause weight loss empowers you with an awareness and appreciation that makes losing weight *and* maintaining your progress attainable.

While many diet books jump right in and give you their diets on page one, the F-Factor Diet is different. In fact, it is the education you gain in the next few chapters that makes the F-Factor Diet unlike any other diet you've tried. You will learn:

- what the food groups are;
- how food gets converted into fat;
- why eating carbohydrates doesn't lead to weight gain; and
- what role fiber plays in your health and in your weight loss.

Understanding these principles will equip you with the necessary tools to begin this program and achieve your health and weight-loss goals.

After patients have lost weight on the F-Factor Diet, many often say, "I owe my weight loss to you." My response is always the same. I say, "I didn't do it; you did. I simply gave you the tools to make your weight loss possible." In order for a person to have achieved his goals, he had to put the tools I gave him to work. A person can thank me for providing the tools but the credit goes to him for applying them. Think of it this way: if I gave you a hammer, nails, and wood, you shouldn't thank me for your house construction. A house will only materialize if the person makes an effort to use the tools and builds a house himself. The same principle applies to dieting.

By applying the tools in the following chapters, you will find that losing weight on the F-Factor Diet is easy to do. The program will simply make sense in a way that no other diet ever has. You will be amazed at how excited you will be to apply the principles you've learned, and you will begin the program with a new insight that will make losing weight a reality.

## Getting Started

Let's begin with a quiz to see how much you know about the fundamentals of nutrition. Grab a pen and take the following quiz:

## Quiz: Is It a Carbohydrate, Protein, or Fat?

All foods are made up of at least one of the major nutrients: carbohydrate, protein, or fat. Each of the foods listed below belongs to one food category: carbohydrate, protein, or fat. Write the name of each food in the circle that shows which food category it belongs to:

| | | |
|---|---|---|
| banana | corn oil | rice |
| potato | salad dressing | bread |
| butter | bagel | cream cheese |
| hamburger patty | egg | macaroni |
| fat-free frozen yogurt | 1% cottage cheese | orange juice |
| corn | tofu | skim milk |
| garbanzo beans | avocado | olive oil |

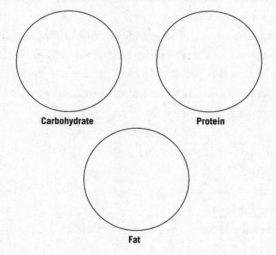

Carbohydrate        Protein

Fat

**ANSWERS:**

**Fat:** corn oil, salad dressing, cream cheese, avocado, olive oil, butter

**Carbohydrate:** banana, rice, potato, bread, bagel, macaroni, fat-free frozen yogurt, orange juice, corn, skim milk, garbanzo beans

**Protein:** hamburger patty, egg, 1% cottage cheese, tofu

**16–21 Correct:** Way to go! You have a good understanding of the food groups.

**8–15 Correct:** You're not quite sure about the food groups. Help's on the way!

**0–7 Correct:** You won't be in the dark for long.

## Nutrition 101: The Food Groups

Many of us grew up with the United States Department of Agriculture's (USDA's) old basic four food groups, first introduced in 1956. The government's basic four involved:

1. protein (meats, poultry, fish, dried beans and peas, eggs, and nuts)
2. dairy (milk, cheese, and yogurt)
3. grains
4. fruits and vegetables

Until 1992, the basic four were a mainstay of nutrition education in the United States and most Americans considered them the definitive word on nutrition. All four groups were assigned equal importance without attention to healthy servings amounts.

In 1992, the USDA issued a food guide pyramid to replace the basic four and to address some of the shortcomings of the old system. Unlike the basic four, the pyramid focused on present health, disease prevention, and the importance of restricting dietary fat. Instead of four food groups, the pyramid created six food groups:

1. starch
2. fruit and fruit juice
3. milk and yogurt
4. nonstarchy vegetables
5. meat and meat substitutes
6. fats

Fruits and vegetables were separated into two distinct groups, and a fat group was created. Other changes included placing cheese into the meat and meat substitute group and moving beans from the meat group into the starch group.

The pyramid emphasized the nutritional importance of foods based on their placement on the food pyramid. Those at the base, like starch, fruits, and vegetables, were meant to be consumed more than foods near the top, like meat, milk, and fats. Unlike the basic four, the pyramid gave recommendations for how many servings of each food group you should eat. For example, the pyramid recommended a daily 6 to 11 servings of foods in the starch category.

But what exactly counts as a serving? Is a serving of cooked pasta ½ cup or 1 cup? In order to standardize portions for each food group, the dietary exchange lists were created. Foods are grouped by their nutritional content. Each serving of a food has about the same amount of carbohydrate, protein, fat, and calories as the other foods on that list. That is why any food on a list can be "exchanged," or traded, for any other food on the same list.

## The Exchange Lists

Despite their original purpose, the exchange lists have become a useful tool for weight loss and are an integral part of the F-Factor Diet. Although the F-Factor Diet does not require counting calories or grams of fat, you will need to keep track of your carbohydrate and fiber intake, and the exchange lists are the tools that will enable you to do so with ease.

On Step 1, you will use the lists to choose which nonstarchy vegetables and protein (from the very lean and lean lists) you want.

On Step 2, you will use the dietary exchange lists to determine which carbohydrates, and how much of each, to add to your diet. That may sound cumbersome, but I assure you it takes much less effort than you may think.

Therefore, the first step of the F-Factor Diet is to learn which foods are carbohydrates and which are not. The F-Factor Diet divides the 6 food groups into 2 groups, carbohydrate and non-carbohydrate. Starch, fruit/fruit juice, and milk/yogurt are carbohydrates and nonstarchy vegetable, meat/meat substitute, and fat are labeled non-carbohydrate.

| THE CARBOHYDRATE GROUPS: | THE NON-CARBOHYDRATE GROUPS: |
|---|---|
| 1. starch | 1. nonstarchy vegetables |
| 2. fruit/fruit juice | 2. meat and meat substitutes |
| 3. milk/yogurt | 3. fats |

Foods on the carbohydrate list are similar because they each contain 15 grams of carbohydrate per exchange, while foods in the non-carbohydrate group contain 0 grams of carbohydrate. In order to better understand these exchange lists, let's take a look at them:

# 1. STARCH LIST

Each item in this list has these values: 15 grams of carbohydrate, 3 grams of protein, 0–1 gram of fat, and 80 calories

|  | Serving Size | Carbs (g) | Fiber (g) |
|---|---|---|---|
| **BREAD** | | | |
| bagel, 4 oz | ¼ (1 oz) | 15 | 1 |
| biscuit, 2½ inches across | 1 | 15 | 1 |
| bread, reduced calorie | 2 slices | 15 | 1 |
| bread, white | 1 slice | 15 | 1 |
| bread, pumpernickel, rye | 1 slice | 15 | 2 |
| bread, whole-wheat | 1 slice | 15 | 2–6 |
| corn bread, 2-inch cube | 1 (2 oz) | 15 | 1 |
| English muffin | ½ | 15 | 1 |
| English muffin, whole-wheat | ½ | 15 | 2 |
| hot dog bun or hamburger bun | ½ | 15 | 1 |
| naan, 8 x 2 inch | ¼ | 15 | 1 |
| pancake, 4 inches across | 1 | 15 | 0 |
| pancake, whole-wheat | 1 | 15 | 2 |
| pita, 6 inches across | ½ | 15 | 1 |
| pita, whole-wheat, 6 inches across | ½ | 15 | 2 |
| roll, plain, small | 1 (1 oz) | 15 | 1 |
| raisin bread, unfrosted | 1 slice | 15 | 1 |
| stuffing, bread (prepared) | ⅓ cup | 15 | 1–2 |
| taco shell, 5 inches across | 2 | 15 | 1 |
| tortilla, corn or flour, 6 inches across | 1 | 15 | 1 |
| tortilla, flour, 10 inches across | ⅓ | 15 | 1 |
| waffle, 4-inch square, reduced-fat | 1 | 15 | 1 |
| **CEREALS AND GRAINS** | | | |
| bran cereals | ½ cup | 15 | 5–14 |
| bulgur | ½ cup | 15 | 4 |
| cereals, cooked | ½ cup | 15 | 2 |
| cereals, unsweetened, ready-to-eat | ¾ cup | 15 | 0–5 |
| cornmeal (dry) | 2½ tbsp. | 15 | 1–2 |

| | Serving Size | Carbs (g) | Fiber (g) |
|---|---|---|---|
| couscous | ⅓ cup | 15 | 1 |
| flour (dry) | 3 tbsp. | 15 | 1 |
| granola, low-fat | ¼ cup | 15 | 1–3 |
| Grape-Nuts | 3 tbsp. | 15 | 3 |
| grits (cooked) | ½ cup | 15 | 1 |
| kasha (cooked) | ½ cup | 15 | 2 |
| millet (cooked) | ⅓ cup | 15 | 2 |
| muesli | ¼ cup | 15 | 2 |
| oats (dry) | ½ cup | 15 | 2 |
| pasta (cooked) | ½ cup | 15 | 1 |
| puffed cereal | 1½ cups | 15 | 1 |
| quinoa (cooked) | ⅓ cup | 15 | 2 |
| rice, white (cooked) | ⅓ cup | 15 | 1 |
| rice, brown (cooked) | ⅓ cup | 15 | 2 |
| shredded wheat | ⅓ cup | 15 | 2 |
| sugar-frosted cereal | ½ cup | 15 | 0–3 |
| wheat germ | ¼ cup | 15 | 4 |

**STARCHY VEGETABLES**

| | | | |
|---|---|---|---|
| baked beans | ⅓ cup | 15 | 4 |
| corn | ½ cup | 15 | 3 |
| corn on cob, 6 in. | 1 long | 15 | 2 |
| French-fried potatoes (oven baked) | 1 cup | 15 | 2 |
| mixed vegetables with corn, peas | 1 cup | 15 | 3 |
| peas, green | ½ cup | 15 | 4 |
| plantain | ⅓ cup | 15 | 0 |
| potato, boiled | ½ cup | 15 | 2 |
| potato, baked with skin | ¼ large (3 oz) | 15 | 3 |
| potato, mashed | ½ cup | 15 | 2 |
| squash, winter (acorn, butternut, pumpkin) | 1 cup | 15 | 4 |
| yam, sweet potato, plain with skin | ½ cup | 15 | 4 |

**CRACKERS AND SNACKS**

| | | | |
|---|---|---|---|
| animal crackers | 8 | 15 | 0 |

| | Serving Size | Carbs (g) | Fiber (g) |
|---|---|---|---|
| chow mein noodles | ½ cup | 15 | 1 |
| crackers, round butter type | 6 | 15 | 0 |
| graham crackers, 2½ in. square | 3 | 15 | 1 |
| matzoh | ¾ oz | 15 | 1 |
| oyster crackers | 20 | 15 | 0 |
| popcorn (popped, no fat added) | 3 cups | 15 | 3 |
| pretzels | ¾ oz | 15 | 0 |
| rice cakes, 4 inches across | 2 | 15 | 0 |
| saltine-type crackers | 6 | 15 | 0 |
| sandwich crackers, cheese or peanut-butter filling | 3 | 15 | 0 |
| snack chips, fat-free or baked (tortilla, potato) | 8 (¾ oz) | 15 | 2 |
| whole-wheat crackers, no fat added | 2–5 (¾ oz) | 15 | 2 |
| **BEANS, PEAS, AND LENTILS** | | | |
| beans and peas (garbanzo, pinto, kidney, split) | ½ cup | 15 | 6 |
| hummus | ⅓ cup | 15 | 2 |
| lima beans | ½ cup | 15 | 5 |
| lentils (cooked) | ½ cup | 15 | 8 |
| miso | 3 tbsp. | 15 | 3 |

## 2. FRUIT LIST

Each item in this list has these values: 15 grams of carbohydrate, 0 grams of protein, 0 grams of fat, and 60 calories

| **FRUIT** | | | |
|---|---|---|---|
| apple, unpeeled, small | 1 (4 oz) | 15 | 3 |
| applesauce, unsweetened | ½ cup | 15 | 1 |
| apples, dried | 4 rings | 15 | 2 |
| apricots, fresh | 4 whole | 15 | 3 |
| apricots, dried | 8 halves | 15 | 2 |
| apricots, canned | ½ cup | 15 | 2 |

| | Serving Size | Carbs (g) | Fiber (g) |
|---|---|---|---|
| banana, small | 1 (4 oz) | 15 | 2 |
| blackberries | 1 cup | 15 | 8 |
| blueberries | ¾ cup | 15 | 5 |
| cantaloupe, small | 1 cup cubes | 15 | 1 |
| cherries, fresh | 12 | 15 | 2 |
| cherries, sweet, canned | ½ cup | 15 | 1 |
| dates | 3 small/1 large | 15 | 2 |
| figs, dried | 2 | 15 | 2 |
| fruit cocktail | ½ cup | 15 | 1 |
| grapefruit, large | ½ | 15 | 2 |
| grapes | 15 | 15 | 1 |
| honeydew melon | 1 slice | 15 | 1 |
| kiwi | 1 | 15 | 3 |
| mandarin oranges, canned | ¾ cup | 15 | 1 |
| mango, small | ½ cup | 15 | 1 |
| nectarine, medium | 1 | 15 | 2 |
| orange, medium | 1 (6½ oz) | 15 | 3 |
| papaya | ½ fruit | 15 | 3 |
| peach, fresh | 1 | 15 | 2 |
| peaches, canned | ½ cup | 15 | 2 |
| pear, large, fresh | ½ (4 oz) | 15 | 4 |
| pears, canned | ½ cup | 15 | 2 |
| pineapple, fresh | ¾ cup | 15 | 2 |
| pineapple, canned | ½ cup | 15 | 1 |
| plums, small | 2 | 15 | 2 |
| raisins | 2 tbsp. | 15 | 1 |
| raspberries | 1 cup | 15 | 8 |
| strawberries | 1¼ cup | 15 | 4 |
| tangerines, small | 2 | 15 | 2 |
| watermelon | 1¼ cup | 15 | 1 |

**FRUIT JUICE, UNSWEETENED**

| | | | |
|---|---|---|---|
| apple juice/cider | ½ cup | 15 | 0 |

| | Serving Size | Carbs (g) | Fiber (g) |
|---|---|---|---|
| cranberry juice cocktail | ⅓ cup | 15 | 0 |
| cranberry juice cocktail, reduced-calorie | 1 cup | 15 | 0 |
| fruit juice blends, 100% juice | ⅓ cup | 15 | 0 |
| grape juice | ⅓ cup | 15 | 0 |
| grapefruit juice | ½ cup | 15 | 0 |
| orange juice | ½ cup | 15 | 0 |
| pineapple juice | ½ cup | 15 | 0 |
| prune juice | ⅓ cup | 15 | 1 |

## 3. MILK LIST

### FAT-FREE AND LOW-FAT MILK

Each item in this list has these values: 12 grams of carbohydrate (count as 15 grams of carbohydrate), 8 grams of protein, 0–3 grams of fat, and 90 calories

| | | | |
|---|---|---|---|
| fat-free milk | 1 cup | 15 | 0 |
| 1% milk | 1 cup | 15 | 0 |
| buttermilk, low-fat or fat-free | 1 cup | 15 | 0 |
| evaporated fat-free milk | ½ cup | 15 | 0 |
| fat-free dry milk | ⅓ cup dry | 15 | 0 |
| soy milk, low-fat or fat-free | 1 cup | 15 | 1 |
| yogurt, fat-free, sweetened w/no-calorie sweetener | ⅔ cup (6 oz) | 15 | 0 |
| yogurt, plain, fat-free | ⅔ cup | 15 | 0 |

### REDUCED-FAT

Each item in this list has these values: 12 grams of carbohydrate (count as 15 grams of carbohydrate), 8 grams of protein, 5 grams of fat, and 120 calories

| | | | |
|---|---|---|---|
| 2% milk | 1 cup | 15 | 0 |
| soy milk | 1 cup | 15 | 2 |
| yogurt, plain reduced-fat | ⅔ cup (6 oz) | 15 | 0 |

**WHOLE MILK**

Each item in this list has these values: 12 grams of carbohydrate (count as 15 grams of carbohydrate), 8 grams of protein, 8 grams of fat, and 150 calories

|  | Serving Size | Carbs (g) | Fiber (g) |
|---|---|---|---|
| whole milk | 1 cup | 15 | 0 |
| evaporated whole milk | ½ cup | 15 | 0 |
| goat's milk | 1 cup | 15 | 0 |
| yogurt, plain, made from whole milk | 1 cup (8 oz) | 15 | 0 |

## 4. NONSTARCHY VEGETABLES LIST

Each item in this list has these values: 5 grams of carbohydrate (count as zero carbohydrate), 2 grams of protein, 0 grams of fat, and 25 calories

| ONE VEGETABLE SERVING EQUALS ½ CUP COOKED OR 1 CUP RAW: | | |
|---|---|---|
| artichoke | 0 | 6 |
| artichoke hearts | 0 | 4 |
| asparagus | 0 | 3 |
| bean (green, wax) | 0 | 2 |
| bean sprouts | 0 | 1 |
| beets | 0 | 2 |
| broccoli | 0 | 2 |
| Brussels sprouts | 0 | 3 |
| cabbage | 0 | 2 |
| carrots | 0 | 3 |
| cauliflower | 0 | 2 |
| celery | 0 | 1 |
| cucumber | 0 | 1 |
| eggplant | 0 | 3 |
| green onions or scallions | 0 | 1 |
| greens (collard, kale, mustard, turnip) | 0 | 2 |
| kohlrabi | 0 | 5 |
| leeks | 0 | 1 |

|  | Carbs (g) | Fiber (g) |
|---|---|---|
| mixed vegetables (without corn, peas) | 0 | 1 |
| mushrooms | 0 | 1 |
| okra | 0 | 2 |
| onions | 0 | 1 |
| pea pods | 0 | 2 |
| peppers | 0 | 2 |
| salad greens | 0 | 1 |
| spinach | 0 | 2 |
| summer squash | 0 | 2 |
| tomato | 0 | 1 |
| tomato sauce | 0 | 2 |
| tomato/vegetable juice | 0 | 1 |
| turnips | 0 | 2 |
| water chestnuts | 0 | 0 |
| watercress | 0 | 0 |
| zucchini | 0 | 1 |

## 5. MEAT AND MEAT SUBSTITUTE LIST

### VERY LEAN MEAT AND SUBSTITUTE LIST

Each item in this list has these values: 0 grams of carbohydrate, 7 grams of protein, 0–1 grams of fat, and 35 calories

One very lean meat exchange is equal to any one of the following items:

|  | Serving Size | Carbs (g) | Fiber (g) |
|---|---|---|---|
| *Poultry:* chicken or turkey (no skin), Cornish hen, no skin | 1 oz | 0 | 0 |
| *Fish:* fresh or frozen cod, flounder, haddock, halibut, trout, lox, tuna fish (fresh or canned in water) | 1 oz | 0 | 0 |
| *Shellfish:* clams, crab, lobster, scallops, shrimp | 1 oz | 0 | 0 |
| *Game:* duck or pheasant (no skin), venison, buffalo, ostrich | 1 oz | 0 | 0 |

| | Serving Size | Carbs (g) | Fiber (g) |
|---|---|---|---|
| *Cheese with 1 gram of fat or less per ounce:* | | | |
| Fat-free or low-fat cottage cheese | ¼ cup | 0 | 0 |
| Fat-free cheese | 1 oz | 0 | 0 |
| *Other:* processed sandwich meats with 1 gram of fat or less per ounce, such as deli thin turkey, ham, and roast beef | 1 oz | 0 | 0 |
| egg whites | 2 | 0 | 0 |
| egg substitute | ¼ cup | 0 | 0 |
| hot dogs or sausage with 1 gram of fat or less per ounce | 1 oz | 0 | 0 |
| lite tofu | 1 oz | 0 | 0 |
| 0% fat plain Greek or Icelandic yogurt | 1 oz | 0 | 0 |

## LEAN MEAT AND SUBSTITUTE LIST

Each item in this list has these values: 0 grams of carbohydrate, 7 grams of protein, 3 grams of fat, and 55 calories

One lean meat exchange equals any one of the following items:

| | | | |
|---|---|---|---|
| *Beef:* USDA select or choice grades of lean beef trimmed of fat, such as round, sirloin, flank steak, tenderloin, roast (rib, chuck, rump), steak (T-bone, porterhouse, cubed), ground round | 1 oz | 0 | 0 |
| *Pork:* lean pork, such as fresh ham; canned, cured, or boiled ham, Canadian bacon, tenderloin, center loin chop | 1 oz | 0 | 0 |
| *Lamb:* roast, chop or leg | 1 oz | 0 | 0 |
| *Veal:* lean chop, roast | 1 oz | 0 | 0 |
| *Poultry:* chicken, turkey (no skin), chicken (white meat, with skin), duck or goose (no skin) | 1 oz | 0 | 0 |
| *Fish:* herring (uncreamed or smoked) | 1 oz | 0 | 0 |
| oysters | 1 oz | 0 | 0 |
| salmon (fresh or canned), catfish | 1 oz | 0 | 0 |
| sardines (canned) | 2 medium | 0 | 0 |
| tuna (canned in oil, drained) | 1 oz | 0 | 0 |

| | Serving Size | Carbs (g) | Fiber (g) |
|---|---|---|---|
| *Game:* goose (no skin), rabbit | 1 oz | 0 | 0 |
| *Cheese:* 1%-fat cottage cheese | ¼ cup | 0 | 0 |
| grated Parmesan | 2 tbsp. | 0 | 0 |
| cheeses with 3 grams of fat or less per ounce | 1 oz | 0 | 0 |
| *Other:* hot dogs with 3 grams of fat or less per ounce | 1½ oz | 0 | 0 |
| Processed sandwich meat with 3 grams of fat or less per ounce such as turkey, pastrami, or kielbasa | 1 oz | 0 | 0 |

## MEDIUM-FAT MEAT AND SUBSTITUTE LIST

Each item in this list has these values: 0 grams of carbohydrate, 7 grams of protein, 5 grams of fat, and 75 calories

One medium-fat meat exchange equals any one of the following items:

| | Serving Size | Carbs (g) | Fiber (g) |
|---|---|---|---|
| *Beef:* most beef products fall into this category (ground beef, meatloaf, corned beef, short ribs, prime grades of meat trimmed of fat, such as prime rib) | 1 oz | 0 | 0 |
| *Pork:* top loin, chop, Boston butt, cutlet | 1 oz | 0 | 0 |
| *Lamb:* rib roast, ground | 1 oz | 0 | 0 |
| *Veal:* cutlet (ground or cubed, unbreaded) | 1 oz | 0 | 0 |
| *Poultry:* chicken (dark meat, with skin), ground turkey or ground chicken, fried chicken | 1 oz | 0 | 0 |
| *Fish:* any fried fish product | 1 oz | 0 | 0 |
| *Cheese:* with 5 grams or less fat per ounce | | | |
| feta | 1 oz | 0 | 0 |
| mozzarella | 1 oz | 0 | 0 |
| ricotta | ¼ cup | 0 | 0 |
| *Other:* egg (high in cholesterol, limit 3 per week) | 1 | 0 | 0 |
| sausage with 5 grams of fat or less per ounce | 1 oz | 0 | 0 |
| tempeh | ¼ cup | 0 | 0 |
| tofu | 4 oz | 0 | 0 |

Each item in this list has these values: 0 grams of carbohydrate, 7 grams of protein, 8 grams of fat, and 100 calories

Remember that these items are high in saturated fat, cholesterol, and calories and may raise blood cholesterol levels if eaten on a regular basis.

One high-fat meat exchange equals any one of the following items:

| | Serving Size | Carbs (g) | Fiber (g) |
|---|---|---|---|
| *Pork:* spareribs, ground pork, pork sausage | 1 oz | 0 | 0 |
| *Cheese:* all regular cheeses, such as American, cheddar, Monterey Jack, Swiss | 1 oz | 0 | 0 |
| *Other:* processed sandwich meats with 8 grams of fat or less per ounce such as bologna, pimento loaf, salami | 1 oz | 0 | 0 |
| sausage, such as bratwurst, Italian, knockwurst, Polish | 1 oz | 0 | 0 |
| hot dog (beef or pork) | 1 | 0 | 0 |
| bacon | 3 slices | 0 | 0 |

## 6. FAT LIST

With the exception of nuts, some seeds and avocado, all the items in this list have these values: 0 grams of carbohydrate, 0 grams of protein, 5 grams of fat, and 45 calories. The values for nuts, seeds and avocado are listed below accordingly.

Fats are divided into three groups based on the main type of fat they contain: monounsaturated, polyunsaturated, or saturated. Monounsaturated and polyunsaturated fats in the foods we eat are linked with good health benefits. Saturated fats are linked with heart disease. In general, one fat exchange is:

- 1 tsp. of regular butter or vegetable oil
- 1 tbsp. of regular salad dressing

### MONOUNSATURATED FAT

| | | | |
|---|---|---|---|
| avocado, medium | 2 slices | 2 | 1 |
| oil (canola, olive, peanut) | 1 tsp. | 0 | 0 |

| | Serving Size | Carbs (g) | Fiber (g) |
|---|---|---|---|
| nuts: almonds, cashews, mixed (50% peanuts), hazelnuts | 6 nuts | 2 | 1 |
| peanuts | 10 nuts | 2 | 1 |
| pecans | 4 halves | 2 | 1 |
| peanut butter, smooth or crunchy | ½ tbsp. | 2 | 1 |
| pistachios | 11 nuts | 2 | 1 |
| sesame seeds | 1 tbsp. | 0 | 0 |
| tahini | 2 tsp. | 0 | 0 |

## POLYUNSATURATED FAT

| | Serving Size | Carbs (g) | Fiber (g) |
|---|---|---|---|
| margarine: stick, tub, or squeeze | 1 tsp. | 0 | 0 |
| mayonnaise, regular | 1 tsp. | 0 | 0 |
| mayonnaise, low-fat | 1 tbsp. | 0 | 0 |
| nuts: walnuts, pecans, Brazil nuts | 4 halves | 2 | 1 |
| oil (corn, safflower, soybean) | 1 tsp. | 0 | 0 |
| salad dressing: regular, reduced-fat | 2 tbsp. | 0 | 0 |
| seeds: pumpkin, sunflower | 1 tbsp. | 0 | 0 |

## SATURATED FAT

| | Serving Size | Carbs (g) | Fiber (g) |
|---|---|---|---|
| bacon, cooked | 1 slice | 0 | 0 |
| butter, stick | 1 tsp. | 0 | 0 |
| butter, whipped | 1 tsp. | 0 | 0 |
| butter, reduced-fat | 1 tbsp. | 0 | 0 |
| coconut, sweetened, shredded | 2 tbsp. | 0 | 0 |
| coconut milk | 1 tbsp. | 0 | 0 |
| cream, half and half | 2 tbsp. | 0 | 0 |
| cream cheese: | | | |
| regular | 1 tbsp. | 0 | 0 |
| reduced-fat | 1½ tbsp. | 0 | 0 |
| shortening or lard | 1 tsp. | 0 | 0 |
| sour cream: | | | |
| regular | 2 tbsp. | 0 | 0 |
| reduced-fat | 3 tbsp. | 0 | 0 |

# Taking a Closer Look at Each List

## The Carbohydrate Groups

**THE STARCH LIST INCLUDES:**
> breads
> cereals
> pasta and grains
> starchy vegetables
> crackers
> snacks
> cooked beans
> peas
> lentils

Note that all the foods on the starch list have a different serving size. For the serving size listed, each food contains 15 grams of carbohydrate and 80 calories. For example, under Bread, you see that white bread has a serving of 1 slice. Therefore, 1 slice of white bread has 15 grams of carbs and 80 calories.

Now look up rice under the cereals and grain category. The serving of rice listed as an exchange is ⅓ cup. Realistically, the average serving of rice is a one-cup portion. So keep in mind that the food exchanges listed are not necessarily the amounts you would typically eat. If you ate only ⅓ cup rice, you would ingest 15 grams of carbs and 80 calories. But if you had a cup of rice, you would multiply those numbers by 3 and end up with 45 grams of carbohydrate and 240 calories. That is how the exchange list works.

**THE FRUIT / FRUIT JUICE LIST**
In general, one fruit exchange is 1 small fresh fruit, ½ cup canned fruit or ¼ cup dried fruit. An exchange of fruit has 15 grams of carbohydrate (just like a starch exchange) and 60 calories. When you look at the fruit exchange lists, you see that the serving sizes vary from fruit to fruit. Typically, the more water and fiber a fruit contains, the larger the serving size on the exchange list. For example, strawberries (high in fiber) have a serving size of 1¼ cup, while raisins have a measly 2 tablespoons serving size for the same 15 grams of car-

bohydrate and 60 calories. I am not saying raisins are bad for you, because all fruits are loaded with vitamins, antioxidants, and fiber. But if you are trying to lose weight, filling up on foods that offer you bigger portions will result in a more satisfying weight-loss plan.

## THE MILK / YOGURT LIST

Most of us grew up with the four food groups where the dairy group consisted of milk, cheese, and yogurt. Yet on the exchange lists, cheese, cream and other dairy fats are noticeably missing. That is because cheese is found on the meat and meat substitute list while cream and other dairy fats are on the fat list. Both milk and yogurt contain protein (8 grams per serving), but they contain considerably more carbohydrate (15 grams per serving), which is why they are on their own list and not grouped with cheese. Cheese, cream, and other dairy fats contain no carbohydrates and therefore are not grouped with milk and yogurt. That is why on Atkins and other high-protein diets where you are told to limit your intake of carbohydrates, you restrict your intake of milk or yogurt but can eat unlimited amounts of cheese and cream. Unfortunately, people who go on those diets usually end up consuming lots of saturated fats from cheese, while missing the opportunity to enrich their diets with low-fat, high-calcium foods like low-fat milk and yogurt.

Looking at the milk/yogurt exchange list, you see that milk and yogurt are broken down into three groups:

- fat-free/low-fat (0–1%)
- reduced-fat (2%)
- whole

Across the board each milk and yogurt group contains 12 grams of carbohydrate and 8 grams of protein. The difference is in the fat and calorie content: fat-free/low-fat contains 0–3 grams of fat and only 90 calories in comparison to whole milk products, which contain 8 grams of fat and 150 calories.

Many people believe incorrectly that whole milk has more vitamins or protein than skim, which is why it is creamier. They think that skim milk is a weaker, watered-down, less vitamin-packed alternative. In fact, skim milk and whole milk contain the same amount of protein and carbohydrate. The only difference is the fat content and therefore the calorie content. The more fat, the more calories.

Another common misconception is that milk and yogurt are considered protein and not carbohydrate. But in fact, 1 cup of milk has virtually the same carbohydrate content as a slice of white bread (15 grams each). Often people say they don't eat carbs, but they eat milk, yogurt, and even fruit. What they really mean is that they don't eat starches like bread, rice, and pasta. Fruit, juice, milk, and yogurt contain the same amount of carbohydrate per serving as a serving of starch; and, if you are going to eat them, you might as well eat starches, too. In essence, there is no difference between the carbohydrate content of an orange and a piece of whole-wheat toast.

According to the dietary exchange lists, foods on the milk/yogurt list contain 12 grams of carbohydrate per exchange (see page 36). For consistency and ease, the F-Factor Diet rounds the 12 grams up to 15 grams of carbohydrates, so that foods on the starch, fruit/fruit juice, and milk/yogurt lists all contain the same number of carbohydrates per serving. This uniformity makes it easy to remember: all foods on the carbohydrate lists contain 15 grams of carbohydrate per serving.

## The Non-carbohydrate Groups:

Now let's take a look at the three non-carbohydrate groups.

### THE NONSTARCHY VEGETABLES LIST

Vegetables contain a minimal amount of carbohydrate per serving: 5 grams of carbohydrate per 1 cup of raw vegetables or ½ cup cooked vegetables. Due to this carbohydrate content, high-protein, low-carbohydrate diets like Atkins often make you limit your intake of vegetables. Carrots, tomatoes, and even onions are all offenders and are to be consumed in moderation.

Yet limiting your vegetable intake is one of the *worst* things you can do if you are trying to lose weight and improve your health. Vegetables contain antioxidants, vitamins, nutrients, and fiber, and relatively few calories. The reason so many people are overweight is *not* because they are sitting around eating too many vegetables. In fact, it is often a *lack* of vegetables in the diet that leads people to fill up on calorie-dense foods. In all my years of counseling overweight patients, *I have never met anyone who has gained weight from eating too much broccoli or too much lettuce.* In fact, when patients began adding more vegetables to their diets, they felt fuller on fewer calories, enabling them to lose weight without feeling hungry.

When I created the F-Factor Diet, I wanted to make eating vegetables as appealing as possible. Therefore, I took the liberty of labeling nonstarch vegetables a non-carbohydrate food, and giving vegetables a zero gram carbohydrate content (see pages 37–38). The reasoning is that patients are more likely to fill up on vegetables when they think of them as a free food. Since I don't want you to limit your intake of nonstarchy vegetables just to keep your carb count down, we'll count these nutrient-rich, weight-loss-friendly foods as having zero carbs. List them as zero-carb foods on your journal pages. (The recipes in Chapter 11 will show both zeroed-out and actual carb counts for dishes that include vegetables, for your information.)

So eat your vegetables! Just keep in mind that the nonstarchy vegetable category excludes beans, corn, peas, plantains, potato, squash, and sweet potato (all found on the starch list).

### THE MEAT AND MEAT SUBSTITUTE LIST

Meat and meat substitutes contain both protein and fat but no carbohydrate. In general, one meat exchange equals 1 ounce of meat, fish, poultry, or cheese. Based on the amount of fat they contain, meats are divided into:

- very lean
- lean
- medium-fat
- high-fat

Whether a meat or meat substitute is very lean or high-fat, the protein is 7 grams per ounce. As the fat content increases from 0 to 1 gram fat per ounce for very lean to 8 grams fat per ounce for high-fat, the calories increase from 35 to 100 calories per ounce. Since the average portion of meat is typically 4 ounces, when you choose cuts that are fattier, you increase your caloric intake by a few hundred calories. Many high-protein diets allow you to eat as much fatty meat as you would like. This guideline is extremely controversial since many studies have concluded that diets high in fat increase the risk factors for cardiovascular disease and cancer. The F-Factor Diet encourages you to select very lean and lean meat lists while eating from the medium-fat and high-fat lists sparingly. Many people think that lean meats include only fish and chicken. You may be pleasantly surprised to see that lean meats include certain cuts of beef, pork, lamb, veal, and low-fat cheese. You do not have to sacrifice flavor or variety. Relying on the leaner choices guarantees fewer calories and less saturated fat in your diet.

**THE FAT LIST**

Fats contain no carbohydrate, and aside from nuts, seeds, and bacon, no protein either.

Fats are divided into three groups based on the main type of fat they contain: monounsaturated, polyunsaturated, or saturated. Monounsaturated and polyunsaturated fats in the foods we eat are linked with good health benefits. Saturated fats are linked with heart disease. When choosing fats, aim for the fats listed on the monounsaturated lists, as they are the most heart healthy. But keep in mind that all fats are high in calories. Both butter (saturated) and olive oil (monounsaturated) contain 135 calories and 15 grams of fat per tablespoon. Just because a fat is unsaturated does not mean you should eat as much of it as you like. Extra calories from fat will still make you fat whether you are eating too much olive oil or too much butter. But since you need some fat in your diet, opt for the unsaturated fats and simply use them in moderation. A little bit of fat at each meal helps to slow down digestion and keep you feeling fuller for a longer period of time than a meal that does not have fat.

So there you have it: the six food groups divided into carbohydrate and non-carbohydrate groups. Rest assured that you do not need to memorize these lists in order to begin the program. Rather, you will use the lists as a guide. Most people are creatures of habit and tend to eat their favorite foods most often. Those are the foods whose exchanges you will end up committing to memory, and the foods you eat less frequently you will look up on the lists.

Now that we know which groups are carbohydrates, it is time to dispel the myth that eating carbohydrates will make you fat.

# DO CARBOHYDRATES MAKE YOU FAT?
## DISPELLING THE MYTH

*All truths are easy to understand once they are discovered;*
*the point is to discover them.*
—GALILEO GALILEI

ONE OF the greatest diet myths is that carbohydrates make you fat. Nothing could be further from the truth. If the only thing you ate all day was one bagel, that bagel would not make you fat. In fact, if all you ate was a bagel, you would be in a caloric deficit and you would most likely lose weight. It's not that carbohydrates make us fat; it's the quantity we eat that packs on the pounds.

If carbohydrates really made us fat, then Italians, many of whom eat pasta every day, or Asians, whose diet is primarily rice based, would be among the fattest people on earth. But they're not. Again, the answer is quantity. Italians eat pasta as a first course—a *primo piatto*—which consists of about 1½ cups or 375 calories. Then they follow that with a *secondi* or main course of lean meat or fish and vegetables. In the United States, on the other hand, we most often eat pasta as our main course. A typical main course serving of pasta in this country is about 4 cups, or 1,000 calories. Big difference!

In the previous chapter you learned which food groups are considered carbohydrates. The next step is to learn how your body digests and stores them. It's this understanding that will make you realize that *it is not carbohydrates themselves that make you fat but rather overeating the wrong kinds.*

All carbohydrates, whether an apple or a dish of ice cream, contain sugar. The sugar found in starch is called maltose, the sugar in fruit and juice is called fructose, and the sugar in milk and yogurt is called lactose. Maltose, fructose, and lactose are all disaccharides. As food is digested, these sugars get broken down further into a single sugar molecule (monosaccharide) called glucose, which is the end product of carbohydrate metabolism. Whether you eat a bagel, an apple, or a cup of yogurt, the end result is glucose.

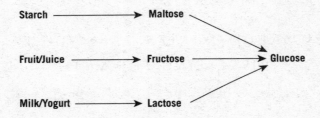

Your body uses glucose to function. In order for glucose to be stored, it must attach itself to a water molecule, $H_2O$. The storage form of glucose is called glycogen. Glycogen gets stored in two places: your liver and your muscles. Your liver is very "generous" with its glycogen stores; the muscles, however, are "selfish" with theirs.

The liver shares its glycogen stores with the heart, brain, and respiratory system. If you've ever seen a movie where a patient is in a coma, there is always a drip attached to his arm. What's in that drip? Glucose. You may think, "If the person is in a coma, why does he need glucose for energy?" The answer is that if he is on a respirator, or if his heart and brain are functioning, he is burning calories. If he did not receive glucose, he would end up depleting his glycogen stores, and then his body would turn to the fat stores for fuel. Once the fat stores are depleted, the body would begin to burn muscle. The heart is a muscle, and eventually the body would break it down for energy. When someone starves to death, he literally ends up using his heart muscles for fuel.

The muscles are very selfish with their glycogen stores. Think of the survival of the fittest, the "fight or flight" syndrome. You always have to have enough stored energy (glycogen) to be able to get up and flee a dangerous environment. Let's say you are reading this book when all of a sudden a fire alarm goes off; you need to have enough stored energy in your muscles to be able to get up and run out of the building. If your muscles shared their glycogen stores with the central nervous system, there would be little glycogen left for physical activity. Then, if the fire alarm went off, the message would quickly get to your brain, but your muscles wouldn't have enough glycogen stored to be able to get you moving out of the room. Therefore, your muscles must keep their glycogen stores for their own personal use.

To review, when you eat carbohydrates, whether in the form of starch, fruit, or milk, they get converted into glucose, which is stored in your muscles and liver as glycogen.

## Tanking Up on Glycogen

Think of your glycogen stores as dual tanks of fuel. One tank is your liver, the other is your muscles, and the fuel is the glycogen.

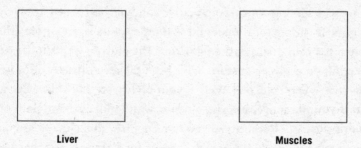

Liver                    Muscles

Okay, here comes the explanation that is going to dispel the myth that carbohydrates make you fat.

Picture the above glycogen stores as a tank of gas in your car. Say you decide to drive cross-country. The first thing you would do is drive to the gas station and fill up the tank with gas, because you know that the more gas you have in the tank, the farther you can drive without stopping to refuel. To apply this idea to the human body, think of a marathon runner. The night before a marathon, runners typically "tank up" by eating a large serving of carbohydrates. This is called carbo-loading. The more carbohydrates runners eat before the race, the more stored glucose (glycogen) or energy they will have. The more stored energy, the farther they can run the next day without having to stop to refuel. Those who take running very seriously even pop glucose tablets as they run. Taking glucose tablets is like driving your car while someone perpetually pumps gas into your tank as you speed along.

So now let's go back to the example of your car and its gas tank. You are back at the gas station, and you decide that you don't want to make any stops between New York and California. You fill the tank up, and once it reaches capacity, you try to put in more gas. What would happen? Clearly the tank would overflow and gas would spill out onto your feet. Most self-service gas stations even have signs warning customers not to "top off" to avoid wasted overflow.

Now let's apply this idea to eating too many carbohydrates. If you start your day with a bagel (6 servings of carbohydrate), have a sandwich (2 pieces of bread, 2 servings carbohydrate), a 1.5-ounce bag of pretzels (2 servings) and an apple (1 serving) for lunch, and a medium-sized frozen yogurt with granola for a snack (3 servings of carbohydrate), you will have filled your glycogen stores. Now it is time for dinner and you order pasta as an entrée. The pasta gets converted into maltose, then glucose. The glucose wants to be stored as glycogen but your glycogen stores have been filled to capacity already. What happens to this extra glucose? Well, if your body were truly like a car, according to the example above the extra glucose would spill over and pour out. But that is not the case. Rather, your body recognizes this glucose as energy. It doesn't want to waste it; it wants to store it for later use. So what happens? Your body converts the surplus glucose into fat and stores it as adipose tissue (body fat) around your body. While your glycogen stores are limited, your fat stores are unlimited. That is why you can get fatter and fatter and fatter from eating too many carbohydrates. The point is that carbohydrates on their own do not make you fat. The excess of what your body can store as glycogen is what makes you fat!

The next logical question then is, "How much carbohydrate can I eat before I get fat?" The answer to that all-important question is what this program is all about. The F-Factor Diet will teach you that magic number and show you which carbs you should choose to ensure that you do not exceed your stores, yet still feel satisfied and energized throughout the day.

## Storage Capacity

The liver has the capacity to store 100 grams of glycogen. The muscles have the capacity to store between 250 and 400 grams of glycogen depending on your muscle mass and physical condition. The average size person stores a total of 350 grams of glycogen per day.

The F-Factor Diet was designed to guarantee that you eat enough carbohydrates for energy but do not exceed what your body can store as glycogen. As a result you get to eat carbohydrates and still lose weight!

## So Do Calories Count?

Absolutely. At the end of the day, it is calories that control weight gain or weight loss. The more calories you eat, the fatter you get. Current diet trends would have you believe that food groups like carbohydrates are to blame for making you fat. As you just learned, however, carbohydrates on their own are not fattening. In fact, both protein and carbohydrates have the same 4 calories per gram. The only way to get fat from eating carbohydrates, or any other food group, is by eating more calories than you burn.

Even the healthiest foods, when eaten in greater amounts than needed for energy, will be stored as fat. For example, if your total energy requirement is 1,800 calories and you eat 2,000 calories from any food (whether it be bread or chicken), you will gain weight. It is not possible to circumvent the laws of thermodynamics and energy balance. Conversely, the only way to lose weight is to take in fewer calories than your body burns.

There are two major reasons the body "burns" calories: 1) to fuel its basal metabolism and 2) to fuel its voluntary activities. Your basal metabolism supports your daily involuntary body functions such as your breathing, your heart's beating, the regulating of your body's temperature, and the sending of nerve and hormonal messages to direct these activities. In a nutshell, your basal metabolic rate (BMR) is the number of calories your body burns at rest to maintain normal body functions every day. That's right, even if you're just sitting on the couch reading this book, your body is burning calories.

There are two steps necessary to determine your daily calorie needs: first, you must calculate your BMR; second, you multiply your BMR by an activity factor.

So what is your BMR? Everyone has a different BMR because height, weight, age, and gender all factor into it. To calculate your BMR, grab a pen and a calculator and follow the steps below.

## Calculating Your Basal Metabolic Rate (BMR)

*For Women*

Harris Benedict Formula[14] for Women:

BMR = 655 + (9.6 × weight in kilos) + (1.8 × height in cm) − (4.7 × age in years)

*For Men*

Harris Benedict Formula for Men:

BMR = 66 + (13.7 × weight in kilos) + (5 × height in cm) − (6.8 × age in years)

*Note:* 2.2 pounds = 1 kilo     1 inch = 2.54 centimeters

*Example:*

You weigh 185 pounds (84 kilos)

You are 5'4" tall (162.5 cm)

You are a 32-year-old woman

Your BMR is 655 + (806) + (291) − (150) = 1,602 calories

## Calculating Your Total Caloric Need

To determine your total daily calorie needs, multiply your BMR by the appropriate activity factor, as follows:

14. The Harris Benedict equation is a formula that uses your BMR and then applies an activity factor to determine your total energy expenditure (calories). The only factor omitted by the Harris Benedict equation is lean body mass. Remember, leaner bodies need more calories than less lean ones. Therefore, this equation will be very accurate in all but the very muscular (will underestimate calorie needs) and the very fat (will overestimate calorie needs).

| ACTIVITY FACTOR | FORMULA TO CALCULATE YOUR BMR |
|---|---|
| Sedentary: little or no exercise | BMR × 1.2 |
| Lightly active: light exercise/sports 1–3 days/week | BMR × 1.375 |
| Moderately active: moderate exercise/sports 3–5 days/week | BMR × 1.55 |
| Very active: very hard daily exercise/sports 6–7 days/week | BMR × 1.725 |
| Extra active: very hard daily exercise/sports/physical job or 2× day training | BMR × 1.9 |

## Your Total Energy Needs: An Example

If your BMR is 1,602, as in the example above, and you are sedentary, you multiply 1602 × 1.2, which equals 1,922. Therefore, your total energy needs are 1,922 calories per day in order to maintain your current weight.

# How Many Calories Do You Need to Lose in Order to Lose Weight?

Once you know the number of calories needed to maintain your weight, you can easily calculate the number of calories you should consume to achieve your weight-loss goal.

To lose weight, you need to create a calorie deficit. There are two ways to do this. The first way is to eat fewer calories than your body burns (BMR). The second way would be to keep your calorie intake the same but increase your activity level so you burn more calories. If you love to exercise and actually have the time to spend hours at the gym, the latter option may work for you. For most people, however, reducing caloric intake is a more realistic option.

There are approximately 3,500 calories in a pound of stored body fat. So, if you create a 3,500-calorie deficit through diet, exercise, or a combination of the two, you will lose one pound of body weight. If you divide the 3,500 calories by 7 days in a week, you get a 500-calorie deficit a day. So if your energy needs for maintenance were 1,922 calories a day, you would need to deduct 500 calories a day.

$$1,922 \text{ calories} - 500 \text{ calories} = 1,422 \text{ calories per day}$$
$$\text{for 1 pound of weight loss a week.}$$

## Don't Let Your Body Think It's Starving

Earlier I explained that your body doesn't want to waste energy. In fact, your body is designed to help you survive in even the most adverse circumstances. If you eat too few calories, your body will think there's a food shortage, and your metabolism will automatically begin to slow down in order to expend as little energy as possible. And you will be tired, irritable, and as a result, totally unmotivated to follow whatever weight-loss plan you are on. The outcome, as you may already have discovered from past diets, is that your weight loss will taper off, or you may stop losing weight entirely.

Many diets promise that you'll shed up to 12 pounds in the first two weeks. If you follow such plans to the letter, that promise might actually come true, but that doesn't mean you're actually losing 12 pounds of body fat. In fact, the average healthy human body simply will not lose more than 2 pounds of fat per week. What you will lose is water, and that's most of what your initial quick weight loss will be—just water.

This is particularly true of high-protein diets that deplete your glycogen stores, because, as I've said, glucose gets stored as glycogen by attaching itself to a water molecule. When the glycogen is burned for energy, the water molecule is released, and some of the weight you lose is water, not body fat.

## The Answer: High-Fiber Carbohydrates

The answer to successful weight loss is to eat fewer calories than you burn without starving yourself. The good news is that you don't have to count calories on the F-Factor Diet. The work has already been done for you. Each step of the F-Factor Diet has a calorie cap that guarantees you will lose weight. You will feel satiated and satisfied, and you need to receive the proper nourishment in order to keep up your energy level and remain in good health. Adding the right amount of high-fiber carbohydrates is the secret to losing weight—easily, painlessly, and for the rest of your life. So what role does fiber play in making your weight-loss goal a reality? The following chapter will give you the answers.

# FIBER: THE SECRET WEAPON FOR HEALTHY WEIGHT LOSS

▬▬ ▬ ▬ ▬ ▬ ▬ ▬ ▬ ▬ ▬ ▬ ▬ ▬ ▬ ▬

*Fiber and protein at every meal*
*Makes losing weight no big deal.*
—TANYA ZUCKERBROT, M.S., R.D.

OKAY, I admit it—fiber isn't sexy. But when it comes to losing weight, nothing is more effective. In fact, a high-fiber eating plan is really the "un-diet"—the one plan that will help you kick those starve-and-cheat, lose-it-and-gain-it-back habits for good, without leaving you hungry. Fiber is one of those nutrients that many of us know is important but that remains a bit of a mystery. Exactly what is it? What are the best sources of fiber? And what are its health benefits? Here you will find answers to all those questions, and by the end of this chapter, you will be ready to begin the F-Factor Diet.

## What Is Fiber?

Basically, fiber is the part of carbohydrates that cannot be digested. Fiber is made up of the tough cell walls of plants that your body can't break down.

Fiber is found in all plant foods including fruits, vegetables, legumes, and grains. Fiber is not found in any animal products, and that includes meat, fish, poultry, eggs, and cheese. The part of the plant fiber that you eat is called dietary fiber and is an important part of any healthy diet.

## Fiber Comes in Two Forms

Dietary fiber comes in two forms: soluble and insoluble.

Soluble fiber swells in your stomach, providing bulk and giving you a feeling of fullness. Good sources of soluble fiber include dried beans and legumes, oatmeal, oat bran, barley, and citrus fruits. Soluble fiber also has cholesterol-lowering properties because it acts like a sponge, absorbing cholesterol and pulling it out of your body.

Insoluble fiber, usually referred to as roughage, includes the woody or structural parts of plants, such as broccoli, apples, wheat bran, and whole-grain cereals. Insoluble fiber tends to speed up the passage of material through the digestive tract and help reduce the risk of colon cancer and diverticular disease. It is often referred to as "nature's broom."

Although you should get both soluble and insoluble fiber in your diet every day, there is no need to fixate on one type or the other. Because most whole plant foods contain both types of fiber, just increasing your intake of foods high in total fiber will provide you with beneficial amounts of both.

### Fiber Facts

- North Americans ate 10 times more fiber 100 years ago than they do today.
- Fiber has zero calories.
- Fiber is only found in carbohydrates. Yet not all carbohydrates contain fiber.
- High-fiber foods provide long-term energy to your body because they are digested and processed more slowly than refined carbohydrates.
- Only 1 in 5 Americans have an idea how much fiber they consume on a daily basis, and only about 22 percent know how many grams of fiber are recommended each day.

## Fiber and Weight Loss Go Hand in Hand

There are many ways to lose weight. In the past, you may have opted to cut out carbohydrates (Atkins), or fat (Dean Ornish), or sugar (Sugar Busters!), or even cooked food (raw foods diet), and succeeded in dropping a few pounds. The problem with all these diets, however, is that they focus on the foods you *can't* eat, which ultimately leaves you feeling deprived, wanting those foods even more.

The difference between the F-Factor Diet and all others is that the F-Factor Diet *requires* you to *add rather than omit food from your diet.* The addition of fiber-rich foods to your diet guarantees that you never feel hungry, making weight loss easier than ever to maintain forever. Not only will you lose weight on the F-Factor Diet, you will also gain improved energy and many other health benefits.

## 1. Fiber Makes Calories Disappear

Yes, you read that right. In fact, a study conducted by David J. Baer of the United States Department of Agriculture's Human Nutrition Research Center in Beltsville, Maryland, found that women who doubled their fiber intake from 12 to 24 grams per day cut their calorie absorption by 90 calories daily. That's a 9.4-pound weight loss in a year!

Another study reported in the *Journal of the American Medical Association* concluded that fiber consumption (or the lack thereof) was more critical than fat consumption for determining future weight gain, blood cholesterol levels, and other risk factors for heart disease.

So how does fiber—which has no nutritional value and simply goes in and comes out—work its magic? The secret is that fiber acts like a sponge in your digestive tract, absorbing other molecules like carbs, fats, and sugars—along with all their calories—and preventing them from settling on your hips. In addition, fiber contributes bulk to foods, which gives you the satisfaction of chewing, plus the feeling of a full stomach, without adding any calories. And since fiber-rich foods take longer to digest, you feel fuller longer, so you tend to eat less throughout the day, making weight loss easy to achieve.

To give you an idea of how fiber works its calorie-reducing magic, let's take a look at two cereals:

## Kellogg's®
## All-Bran®
## Original

| Nutrition Facts | | |
|---|---|---|
| Serving Size | | ½ Cup (31g) |

| Amount Per Serving | Cereal | with ½ cup skim milk |
|---|---|---|
| **Calories** | 80 | 120 |
| Calories from Fat | 10 | 10 |

| | | % Daily Value** | |
|---|---|---|---|
| **Total Fat** 1g* | | 2% | 2% |
| Saturated Fat 0g | | 0% | 0% |
| *Trans* Fat 0g | | | |
| Polyunsaturated Fat 0.5g | | | |
| Monounsaturated Fat 0g | | | |
| **Cholesterol** 0mg | | 0% | 0% |
| **Sodium** 80mg | | 3% | 6% |
| **Potassium** 350mg | | 10% | 16% |
| **Total Carbohydrate** 23g | | 8% | 10% |
| Dietary Fiber 10g | | 40% | 40% |
| Sugars 6g | | | |
| **Protein** 4g | | | |

## Sunbelt Bakery®
## Low-Fat Granola
## Whole Grain Cereal

| Nutrition Facts | |
|---|---|
| Serving Size 1/2 Cup (56g) | |
| Servings Per Container About 8 | |

| Amount Per Serving | |
|---|---|
| **Calories** 220    Calories from Fat 25 | |

| | % Daily Value* |
|---|---|
| **Total Fat** 3g | 5% |
| Saturated Fat 0.5g | 3% |
| Trans Fat 0g | |
| Polyunsaturated Fat 1g | |
| Monounsaturated Fat 1.5g | |
| **Cholesterol** 0mg | 0% |
| **Sodium** 60mg | 3% |
| **Potassium** 170mg | 5% |
| **Total Carb.** 44g | 15% |
| Dietary Fiber 3g | 12% |
| Sugars 17g | |
| **Protein** 5g | |

First, the amount of fiber is part of the total amount of carbohydrates listed on these labels, but since fiber isn't digestible, you get to deduct it from the amount of carbohydrate you're eating.

Kellogg's All-Bran Original cereal, as you can see, has 23 grams of carbohydrate and 10 grams of fiber per ½ cup serving. To determine the *digestible amount* of carbohydrate (net carbohydrate), you subtract the fiber from the total carbohydrate listed on the label.

23 g total carbohydrate – 10 g fiber = 13 g digestible carbohydrate
(net carbohydrate)

By comparison, the same serving size of granola (½ cup) contains 44 grams of carbohydrate and only 3 grams of fiber.

44 g total carbohydrate – 3 g fiber = 41 g digestible carbohydrate

You are getting 28 grams more of digestible carbohydrate from the granola than from the All-Bran cereal because of the lack of fiber in the granola. Since all digestible carbohydrate gets converted into glucose and stored as glycogen, the extra 28 grams in the granola will fill up your "tank" (glycogen stores) more quickly and therefore leave less room for more carbohydrates later in the day. When your glycogen tank is full, any excess carbohydrate cannot be stored as glycogen and will be converted into fat and stored as fat. That's why you should aim for foods with the most fiber: *the more fiber a food contains, the less digestible carbohydrate your body stores!*

But that is not the only benefit. The more fiber in a food, the fewer calories it contains. For the same ½ cup of cereal, the low-fiber granola contains 220 calories while the All-Bran Original cereal contains only 80 calories. That's a difference of 140 calories for the exact same portion size. If 140 calories doesn't seem like very much, just remember that 3,500 calories equals 1 pound of body fat. So if you did nothing except eat the granola for breakfast instead of the All-Bran Original every morning for a year, you'd have consumed an additional 51,100 calories, which translates to almost 15 pounds of weight gain in those 12 months.

Nutrition is a science. So, as in mathematics, the numbers have to add up. To see this, let's return to the exchange lists in Chapter 3.

When we look at the starch list, it shows that every serving of starch contains 15 grams of carbohydrate and 80 calories.

> 15 grams carbohydrate = 80 calories

If you add another serving, you get:

> 30 grams carbohydrate = 160 calories

Add still another serving, and you get:

> 45 grams carbohydrate = 240 calories, and so on.

The more carbohydrate, the more calories.

All-Bran Original contains 13 grams net carbs, which is less than 15 grams, so it should logically have no more than 80 calories. And it does. Look at the label; you'll see All-Bran Original has 80 calories per serving.

The granola has 41 grams net carbs, which should give it between 160 calories and 240 calories (see page 62). The granola has 220 calories—almost three times the calories in the All-Bran Original for the same ½ cup portion.

You can see that the fiber content makes a *drastic* difference not only in the net carbs but also in the *caloric content* of the two cereals. I chose a low-fat granola. There are only 3 grams of fat. The calories are from the *carbs*.

The good news is the F-Factor Diet does not force you to count calories. That does not mean, however, that calories don't count. Of course they do. In fact, it's too many calories from all foods that pack on the pounds. The reason you don't have to count calories on the F-Factor Diet is that there is a calorie cap built into the program. As long as you reach your fiber goal, limiting your intake of simple carbohydrates to the amount allowable in each step, you are guaranteed to feel full without exceeding your calorie needs for the day.

## 2. A High-Fiber Diet Improves Your Energy Throughout the Day

Do you ever feel ravenous only hours after a big meal? Do you find yourself crashing at work in the late afternoon and heading to the vending machine for a pick-me-up? Feelings of fatigue, crankiness, shakiness, and sluggishness can all be symptoms of low blood sugar. After you eat a meal with carbohydrates, your serum glucose levels spike, giving you a sensation of quick energy. But if that meal contains simple carbohydrates (carbs without fiber), you will find yourself crashing soon after.

Simple carbohydrates, such as rye bread and pound cake, usually have a high glycemic index. The glycemic index is a ranking of carbohydrates based on their immediate effect on blood glucose (blood sugar) levels. It compares foods gram for gram of carbohydrate. Carbohydrates that break down quickly during digestion have the highest glycemic indexes. The blood glucose response is fast and high. Carbohydrates that break down slowly, releasing glucose gradually into the bloodstream, have low glycemic indexes. Protein and fat do not raise blood glucose directly and, therefore, do not have a glycemic index; however, these foods, like fiber, slow digestion.

By eating a combination of fiber and protein at every meal, you are providing your body with long-term energy. Your sugars will not spike, nor will they crash, thus guaranteeing an even, well-balanced level of energy throughout the day. If there is one thing my patients notice right away, it is that by increasing their fiber intake, they have much more energy all day long.

## Boost Your Daily Fiber

The typical American diet contains no more than 15 grams of fiber per day. By making a few easy switches, you can easily increase your fiber intake without sacrificing flavor or fullness.

| TYPICAL DAY | HEALTHY FIBER DAY |
| --- | --- |
| **Breakfast** | |
| fried eggs, 2 | egg white (4) omelet with spinach |
| white toast with butter, 1 slice | whole-wheat toast, 1 slice |
| cornflakes (1 cup) with milk | All-Bran Bran Buds (⅓ cup) with skim milk |
| orange juice, 1 cup | 1 orange, sliced into wedges |
| coffee | coffee |
| **Lunch** | |
| tomato soup (1 cup) | lentil soup (1 cup) |
| turkey sandwich on white bread with mayonnaise | turkey sandwich on whole-wheat bread with lettuce, tomato, and mustard |
| 2 chocolate chip cookies | 2 oatmeal raisin cookies |
| **Snack** | |
| potato chips, 1 oz | 2 cups low-fat popcorn |
| **Dinner** | |
| fried chicken, 2 pieces | grilled chicken breast |
| mashed potato (1 cup) with butter | baked potato with skin |
| white roll | whole-grain roll |
| ½ ear corn | 1 cup broccoli |
| ice cream (1 cup) with chocolate sauce (1 tbsp.) | strawberries (1 cup) with chocolate sauce (1 tbsp.) |
| **Total** | **Total** |
| Calories: 2,640 | Calories: 1,470 |
| Carb: 303 g | Carb: 232 g |
| Fiber: 12 g | Fiber: 45 g |
| Fat: 117 g | Fat: 25 g |

# Health Effects of Eating Fiber

If you saw a food label that said, "May reduce the risk of heart disease, diabetes, cancer, could lower your cholesterol and control your appetite," you would think it was a scam. Yet that is exactly what fiber does. Adding fiber-rich foods to your diet is one of the best things you can do to increase your chances for a long and healthy life.

## 1. Fiber protects against heart disease.

About 84 million Americans are living with some form of cardiovascular disease (CVD), the single leading cause of death in the United States. A person's levels of blood lipids—HDL and LDL cholesterol as well as triglycerides—provide a good gauge of heart health. The lower your LDL and triglyceride levels, the less likely you are to develop heart disease.

In an effort to lower their cholesterol and risk of CVD, Americans often choose the easy road and turn to medication rather than change their diet. Statins (cholesterol-lowering medications) drive a $29-billion-a-year worldwide market, with Lipitor number one—of *all* prescription drugs—in retail sales in the U.S.

The number-one dietary change that a person can make in order to improve his or her cholesterol is to eat more fiber. Fiber helps to lower cholesterol by binding with cholesterol in the gastrointestinal tract and ushering it out of the body before it has a chance to reach the bloodstream, where it would otherwise clog up arteries. Thousands of patients on the F-Factor Diet have seen amazing improvements in their cholesterol levels in just eight weeks on the program. Patients once on statin drugs were able to reduce their dosage and in some cases discontinue taking the medication altogether. Achieving a desirable cholesterol level is one of the best ways to reduce the risk for cardiovascular disease, including heart attack and stroke.

## 2. Fiber decreases the risk for diabetes.

Diabetes is becoming one of the fastest-growing diseases in this country. Roughly 30 million Americans have diabetes and another 84 million people have prediabetes (people with prediabetes have blood sugar levels that are

## A Primer on Blood Lipids

High cholesterol affects 28.5 million Americans, and 94.6 million more have borderline high cholesterol. Cholesterol, which is a waxy substance produced by the liver and supplied by animal foods, is tested with a simple blood test that measures the total amount of cholesterol in your blood. Everyone age twenty and older should have his or her cholesterol measured at least once every five years. It is best to have a blood test called a "lipoprotein profile" to find out cholesterol numbers. This blood test is done after a 9- to 12-hour fast and gives information about:

- Your total cholesterol
  Desirable—less than 200 mg/dL
  Borderline high risk—200–239 mg/dL
  High risk—240 mg/dL and over

- Your LDL (bad) cholesterol—the main source of cholesterol buildup and blockage in the arteries
  Optimal—less than 100 mg/dL
  Optimal/above optimal—100–129 mg/dL
  Near borderline high—130–159 mg/dL
  High—160–189 mg/dL
  Very high—190 mg/dL and above

- Your HDL (good) cholesterol—helps keep cholesterol from building up in the arteries
  Low—less than 40 mg/dL
  Average level for men—40–50 mg/dL
  Average level for women—50–60 mg/dL
  Desirable—above 60 mg/dL

- Your triglycerides—another form of fat in the blood
  Normal—less than 150 mg/dL
  Borderline high—150–199 mg/dL
  High—200–499 mg/dL
  Very high—500 mg/dL or higher

> **Helpful hint:**
>
> Here's an easy way to remember your levels when you get your cholesterol checked:
>
> - You want your **H**DL to be "**H**igh" and your **L**DL to be "**L**ow."
>
> I recommend having a cholesterol screening before beginning this program. If you have elevated cholesterol levels, the program will help you to lower your LDL and triglycerides. After eight weeks on the F-Factor Diet, get another cholesterol screening and you'll be amazed at the improvement in your cholesterol.

higher than normal but not high enough to be diabetic). If people with pre-diabetes lose weight and exercise, they can delay or even prevent diabetes altogether.

The F-Factor Diet not only enables weight loss but also helps to control blood sugars throughout the day. Studies have shown that people who eat a high-fiber diet lowered their risk of diabetes by 30 percent.[15]

## 3. Fiber decreases the risk for breast cancer.

Breast cancer incidence in women has increased from 1 in 20 in 1960 to 1 in 8 today and is the leading cancer among white and African American women. Recent studies have shown a strong correlation between a high-fiber diet and a reduced risk factor for breast cancer.

As reported in the *Journal of Clinical Oncology* (July 2004) researchers found that a diet including 20 to 30 grams of fiber per day can lower blood estrogen levels. Estrogen stimulates the early growth and development of breast cancer. Therefore, the less estrogen you have in your body, the lower your cancer risk. A groundbreaking study led by researchers at Harvard's T.H. Chan School of Public Health, published in *Pediatrics* (February 2016), found that

15. M. Franz, J. Bantle, C. Beebe, et al., "Evidence-based Nutrition Principles and Recommendations for the Treatment and Prevention of Diabetes and Related Complications" (American Diabetes Association position statement), *Journal of the American Dietetic Association* 102, no.1 (January 2002): 109–18.

a high-fiber intake during adolescence was associated with a 16 percent lower risk of overall breast cancer and a 24 percent lower risk of breast cancer before menopause. For each additional ten grams of fiber intake daily during early adulthood, breast cancer risk dropped by 13 percent. These findings suggest it's never too early for young women to embrace a high-fiber diet.[16]

Research into the effects of fiber on the risk of breast cancer is still in the early stages. Yet, considering that 1 in 8 women alive today will get this disease, and one-third of these women will die from it, adding fiber to your diet now is a smart move.

## 4. Fiber reduces blood pressure.

High blood pressure, or hypertension, is called the silent killer because the majority of those who suffer from it have no symptoms. About 1 in 5 Americans have high blood pressure—defined as blood pressure above 140/90. High blood pressure afflicts 50 percent of people aged 55 to 65 and, if left unchecked, results in strokes, heart failure, heart attacks, and death. High blood pressure contributes to half a million strokes and to over a million heart attacks each year.

Recent research reveals that eating a high-fiber diet can reduce elevated blood pressure. In a study conducted at Tulane University, researchers found that getting an extra 7 to 19 grams of fiber a day cut systolic pressure (the upper number) by an average of 5.95 points and diastolic pressure (the lower number) by 4.2 points in eight weeks. Fiber reduces insulin resistance—a suspected step in developing high blood pressure—and inhibits weight gain—a known hypertension risk factor.

## 5. Fiber increases elimination and protects against colon cancer.

Excluding skin cancers, colon cancer is the third most common cancer diagnosed in men and women in the United States and the second leading cause of cancer-related deaths. Studies have shown that a high intake of dietary fiber is associated with a lower risk of colon cancer. Diets high in fiber (30 grams or more) have been shown to reduce the risk of colon cancer by 40 percent.

16. "Dietary Fiber Intake in Young Adults and Breast Cancer Risk," Maryam S. Farvid, A. Heather Eliassen, Eunyoung Cho, Xiaomei Liao, Wendy Y. Chen, and Walter C. Willett, online February 1, 2016, *Pediatrics* 137(3):e20151226 doi: 10.1542/peds.2015-1226.

Harvard University researchers found that butyrate, a fermentation breakdown product of fiber, induces the expression of p21, a tumor suppressor gene in colon cancer cells that causes them to cease growing.[17]

Fiber seems to fight colon cancer by binding to or diluting carcinogens in the gut and speeding them through the colon. These days, it's almost impossible to avoid the toxins in our food supply. We're constantly warned against the mercury in fish, the nitrites in bacon and other smoked meats, and the pesticide residue in chicken, to name just a few of the potential food-based health challenges we face. So getting them out of our system before they can cause damage is one of the things we can do to protect ourselves. In addition, regular elimination is, by itself, beneficial to health.

## 6. High-fiber diets alleviate constipation.

Constipation is defined as a condition in which you have fewer than three bowel movements per week, and is one of the most common gastrointestinal complaints in the United States. Last year more than 4 million people reported suffering frequent constipation, and sales of laxatives exceeded $1.3 billion. The inherent danger of laxatives is that when they're overused, or when used over a long term, they can cause a laxative dependency. The abuse of laxatives is usually not intentional. It may simply start with the use of a stimulant laxative to achieve overnight relief from constipation. If an individual has been coping with constipation for some time, however, the relief from constipation can feel profound and may be enough to inspire further use (or abuse) of laxatives.

People who take laxatives regularly can become dependent upon them for movement of their bowels, requiring ever-increasing dosages to achieve the desired effect until finally the intestine becomes insensitive and fails to work properly. Frequent use of laxatives can induce constipation as the tissues of the colon lining become dried out, muscles are weakened, and nerves are damaged. This breakdown in normal colon functions slows intestinal motility and results in constipation, the very condition one initially intended to remedy

17. E. J. Jacobs and E. White, "Constipation, Laxative Use, and Colon Cancer Among Middle-aged Adults," *Epidemiology* 9 (July 1998): 385–91.

with the laxative use. Because laxatives overempty the bowel, another bowel movement may not occur for as long as three days or more. By the third day, anxiety over failure to move the bowels can lead to the decision to take another dose of laxatives, which further empties the bowel. This is often the start of a cycle of frequent laxative use and, ultimately, laxative abuse.

The number one way to avoid constipation is to eat a diet rich in fiber. Fiber is made up of the tough cell walls of plants that your body cannot break down. Fiber is basically indigestible, leading it to be expelled in the feces. The more fiber you eat, the more you increase stool bulk. Firm, well-formed stools lead to easy, regular defecation. The F-Factor Diet, with its 35 grams of fiber a day deriving from fruits, vegetables, and whole grains, promises to alleviate constipation once and for all.

## What Is Your Fiber Goal and How Do You Reach It?

On the F-Factor Diet, you will be eating at least 35 grams of fiber a day. The American Dietetic Association recommends 20 to 25 grams for the general population and 30 to 40 grams for people with cholesterol levels in excess of 200. The National Academy of Science found that 90 percent of Americans don't meet their recommended daily intake of fiber.

In fact, most Americans consume no more than 10 to 15 grams of fiber per day. Given that figure, reaching your goal may seem a bit overwhelming, but I promise you that it isn't. To the contrary, the F-Factor Diet ensures your success. On Step 1, which you'll be following for two weeks to jump-start your weight loss, you are required to eat 3 servings of high-fiber carbohydrates every day: a high-fiber cereal (13 g fiber), up to 8 high-fiber crackers (32 g fiber), plus 1 piece of high-fiber fruit (4 g fiber) equals 49 grams of fiber.

Then, on Step 2, which you'll follow until you reach your weight-loss goal, you'll have the opportunity to add even more high-fiber carbohydrates. So don't let 35 grams a day scare you. You may be surprised at how easily it all adds up. Below is a sample menu for an average day on Step 2, showing how simple and delicious adding fiber to your diet can be.

# Sample Day on Step 2

BREAKFAST:

Berry Parfait (layers of cottage cheese, All-Bran Bran Buds cereal, blueberries), and iced coffee

*Total Fiber for Breakfast: 18 grams*

| FOOD | SERVING | FIBER |
| --- | --- | --- |
| high-fiber cereal | ⅓ cup | 13 grams |
| blueberries | ¾ cup | 5 grams |
| cottage cheese | 1 cup | 0 grams |
| iced coffee | 1 cup | 0 grams |

LUNCH:

Roasted turkey sandwich on toasted whole-wheat bread with lettuce, tomato, 2 slices avocado, and mustard, and 8 ounces unsweetened iced raspberry tea

*Total Fiber for Lunch: 8 grams*

| FOOD | SERVING | FIBER |
| --- | --- | --- |
| whole-wheat bread | 2 slices | 6 grams |
| sliced turkey breast | 4 ounces | 0 grams |
| lettuce, tomato, avocado | 2 pieces lettuce, 2 slices each tomato and avocado | 2 grams |
| unsweetened iced tea | 8 ounces | 0 grams |

SNACK:

2 high-fiber crackers with 2 tablespoons peanut butter, and a decaf cappuccino

*Total Fiber for Snack: 10 grams*

| FOOD | SERVING | FIBER |
| --- | --- | --- |
| fiber crackers | 2 crackers | 8 grams |
| peanut butter | 2 tablespoons | 2 grams |
| cappuccino | 8 ounces | 0 grams |

**DINNER:**

5 ounces filet mignon, 1 cup baked sweet potato fries, and 1 cup sautéed garlic spinach

*Total Fiber for Dinner: 8 grams*

| FOOD | SERVING | FIBER |
| --- | --- | --- |
| filet mignon | 5 ounces | 0 grams |
| baked sweet potato fries | 1 cup | 4 grams |
| sautéed garlic spinach | 1 cup | 4 grams |

*Total Daily Fiber Intake: 44 grams*

## Can I Get Fiber from Supplements, Drinks, or Pills?

While fiber supplements and drinks are useful for promoting regularity, they have not shown the same calorie-repelling effect as whole foods. Many of the popular diets (including Atkins and South Beach) recommend that you take Metamucil to alleviate constipation, which often accompanies a high-protein diet. Constipation occurs because you are cutting back on carbohydrates, and since fiber is found only in carbohydrates, it is virtually impossible for you to meet your fiber needs on these diets.

The F-Factor Diet does not recommend taking fiber supplements as a replacement for fiber-rich foods. When you get fiber from foods, you also tap into the vitamins, minerals, and phytonutrients (substances found in plant foods that help fight cancer and cardiovascular disease) that come along for the ride. Experts believe that it is the synergy of all these nutrients, most of which aren't contained in fiber supplements, that promotes the most dramatic health benefits. And best of all, because your goal is to get 30 to 38 grams of fiber a day on the F-Factor Diet, you will have enough fiber in your diet to make constipation a thing of the past.

After reading this chapter, you are now ready to begin the F-Factor Diet and make the transition from eating the typical American low-fiber fare to consuming a diet that is natural, rich in nutrients, satisfying, and delicious. On the F-Factor Diet you eat meals that are nourishing and filling, and that give you more energy than ever before. And the best part of it all is that you will be losing fat from day one and keeping it off with minimal effort.

## Quick Overview of the F-Factor Diet

You're probably eager to get started with your new weight-loss program. So here's a brief overview of the steps you'll read about and follow in Chapters 6 to 8.

### Step 1: Jump-start Your Weight Loss

The first two weeks of this program consists of a high-protein, low-fat diet with a moderate amount of high-fiber foods. Step 1 is designed to jump-start your weight loss and give you the confidence that this plan works. If it is followed *exactly* (no cheating), you can lose four to six pounds in the first two weeks.

The only carbohydrates allowed on Step 1 are: All-Bran Original, or All-Bran Bran Buds, Fiber One, or Nature's Path SmartBran cereal, high-fiber crackers, such as GG Bran Crispbreads (up to 8 a day), and one serving of fresh fruit per day. The good news is that you can eat unlimited protein from the very lean and lean exchange lists and generous portions of vegetables from the nonstarchy vegetable list. You are also allowed some healthy fat, like a serving of nuts for a snack, or some olive oil on your salad.

Keeping daily journals will guide you to meet your goals of at least 35 grams fiber and less than 35 grams net carbohydrate a day.

### Step 2: Continued Weight Loss

Step 2 adds three servings of carbohydrates into Step 1. Your goal on Step 2 is to keep *digestible* carbohydrate intake below 75 grams per day while still aiming for at least 35 grams of fiber a day.

By now you should have a good understanding as to which foods contain carbohydrate and which don't. On Step 2, you decide what carbohydrates you want to add back into your diet. You have three servings to play with. You can combine all three servings of carbohydrates for one meal (i.e., 1 cup of rice with dinner) or divide them into three meals (one serving of carbohydrate at breakfast, lunch, and dinner). You decide!

Missing fruit? Now is the time to add another piece into your diet each day. Do you miss bread? Step 2 allows you to have a sandwich. Adding a piece of fruit (15 grams carbohydrate) and a sandwich (made with two slices of bread, 30 grams carbohydrate) would equal your three servings (or 45 grams added carbohydrate). As long as you do not exceed adding more than 45 grams of carbohydrate from an item, you can eat any food and still continue to lose weight.

You will learn to read food labels and calculate how much of the package you are entitled to eat for your serving of carbohydrate (one serving = 15 grams of carbohydrate). It is important that you use the exchange lists included in this book. The exchange lists will help you to become familiar with the correct portion size of the carbohydrates you chose.

## SOME SURPRISING SOURCES OF FIBER

| | Fiber (g) | | Fiber (g) |
|---|---|---|---|
| FRUIT | | whole-wheat | |
| apple | 4 g | spaghetti (1 cup) | 6 g |
| avocado (1 medium) | 8 g | | |
| blackberries (1 cup) | 8 g | BEANS/NUTS | |
| blueberries (¾ cup) | 5 g | BEANS AND PEAS, 1 CUP: | |
| dried figs (3) | 3 g | black-eyed peas | 8 g |
| pear | 5 g | great northern beans | 12 g |
| raspberries (1 cup) | 8 g | lentils or split peas | 15 g |
| strawberries (1¼ cup) | 4 g | pinto or black beans | 10 g |
| | | kidney beans | 14 g |
| VEGETABLES | | garbanzo beans | |
| artichoke, 1 large | 9 g | (chickpeas) | 13 g |
| carrots, ½ cup cooked | 3 g | | |
| collard greens, ½ cup cooked | 2 g | NUTS, 1 OUNCE: | |
| baked potato, with skin | 4 g | almonds, | |
| corn, 1 ear | 4 g | approx. 24 | 4 g |
| spinach, 1 cup cooked | 4 g | peanut butter, 2 tbsp. | 2 g |
| | | pecans, approx. | |
| GRAINS & CEREALS | | 15 halves | 3 g |
| barley, ½ cup cooked | 3 g | walnuts, approx. | |
| popcorn (3½ cups) | 4 g | 14 halves | 4 g |

|  | Fiber (g) |  | Fiber (g) |
|---|---|---|---|
| PRODUCTS | | Surkin Fiber Syrup and | |
| Dannon Oikos Triple Zero | | Honey Alternative | 28 g |
| Greek nonfat yogurt | 6 g | Lily's Sweets dark chocolate | |
| New Pop Skinless Popcorn | 4 g | premium baking chips (5) | 4 g |
| Enlightened Ice Cream bars | 5 g | ChocoRite Chocolate Crispy | |
| F-Factor Fiber/Protein Bar | 20 g | Caramels (1 package) | 13 g |
| Thomas' English muffin light | | | |
| multigrain (1 muffin) | 8 g | | |

Remember:

1 serving = 15 g carbohydrate

2 servings = 30 g carbohydrate

3 servings = 45 g carbohydrate

You will remain on step 2 until you reach your desired weight. Continue to keep a daily journal to monitor your net carbohydrate and fiber intake. On step 2 your goal for fiber remains the same (minimum 30 to 35 grams per day), but the added 45 grams of carbohydrate allows you 75 grams or less net carbohydrate intake.

## Step 3: Maintaining Your Desired Weight

When you have reached your desired weight, you'll begin step 3. Step 3 incorporates three more servings of carbohydrates into Step 2 for a total of 6 additional servings of carbohydrates per day (an additional 45 grams added to Step 2). Your net carbohydrate intake on Step 3 will be less than 125 grams per day (on average), with a continued fiber intake of at least 35 grams per day.

Step 3 is the maintenance phase. You'll never go off Step 3. By now, you have a new way of eating that enables you to eat plenty of fresh fruits and vegetables, lots of lean protein and dairy, and even moderate amounts of fat. You'll also eat carbohydrates, but you will find that you gravitate to carbohydrates that contain fiber because of all the health benefits and the role fiber plays in weight loss. Eating foods high in fiber is what enabled you to lose weight without feeling hungry. You will have a new outlook on food, and you won't feel deprived.

# The Top 10 Fiber Myths Debunked

**1. MYTH:** Fiber tastes terrible.

**REALITY:** Until recently, fiber may have brought to mind dry, tasteless bran products that are hard to swallow. The truth is that fiber is found in many delicious foods including fresh fruit, crunchy vegetables, nuts, cereals, breads, pasta, and legumes. Food companies are also jumping on the high-fiber bandwagon and have introduced delicious fiber-rich items to the marketplace including yogurt, chocolate, snack bars, cookies, crackers, and even orange juice. Never has it been so easy, or so delicious, to eat a high-fiber diet.

**2. MYTH:** Since fiber is only found in carbohydrates, won't eating all these carbohydrates cause weight gain?

**REALITY:** No. While eating too many carbohydrates can lead to weight gain, fiber is the secret to eating carbohydrates and shedding pounds. Fiber is the zero-calorie, indigestible component of carbohydrates. The more fiber a food contains, the less digestible carbohydrate (net carbohydrate) there is. It is the net carbohydrate, not the total carbohydrate, that gets converted into glucose. If you have too much glucose, the excess gets converted into fat and stored as fat. High-fiber carbohydrates have lower net carbohydrate than foods that contain no fiber. In addition, fiber adds texture, bulk, and chewing satisfaction, which aids in consuming fewer calories yet still feeling full. The longer you feel full after a meal, the less likely you are to overeat later on, leading ultimately to weight loss. Fiber is truly a dieter's secret weapon.

**3. MYTH:** Salads are a great source of fiber.

**REALITY:** Many people falsely believe that lettuce and salads are a good source of fiber. The truth is lettuce contains very little fiber, approximately 1 gram per cup.

| LETTUCE, 1 CUP | FIBER |
| --- | --- |
| iceberg | .70 g |
| romaine | .95 g |
| radicchio | .36 g |
| arugula | .32 g |
| Bibb, Boston, butter | .55 g |
| endive | 1.55 g |

Although lettuce itself isn't a high-fiber food, a mixed salad filled with beans and vegetables is a great way to get fiber in your diet. Think of lettuce as the foundation, and add other fiber-rich vegetables and legumes to it. Add ½ cup of garbanzo beans, ½ cup of broccoli, a few carrots and slices of red pepper, and you just increased the fiber content by approximately 10 grams!

What Grandma calls "roughage" scientists call "fiber." Roughage and fiber are both terms used to describe the indigestible part of carbohydrates found in plant foods such as fruits, vegetables, and whole grains.

Many people mistakenly believe that all vegetables are roughage and therefore contain large amounts of fiber. The reality is that not all vegetables are good sources of fiber. For example, broccoli, asparagus, and spinach are all good sources of fiber, while lettuce, cucumbers, and celery have very little fiber. Don't assume that just because a food is a vegetable it contains a lot of fiber.

**4. MYTH:** All fruits are good sources of fiber.
**REALITY:** While all fruits contain some fiber, some pack a bigger punch than others. Fruits you eat with the skin on, like apples and pears, tend to have more fiber than fruits that you peel (oranges and bananas). Fruits with seeds are filled with fiber, which makes raspberries, strawberries, blueberries, figs, and blackberries all great choices. While dried fruit is a good source of fiber, be careful with the quantity since they pack a lot of calories and are sometimes sold in sugar-added varieties. Canned fruits have the least amount of fiber since they are peeled and processed, so stick with fresh fruit whenever possible.

**5. MYTH:** It is impossible to get enough fiber from foods alone. Fiber supplements like powders and pills are a great way to get my daily fiber requirement.
**REALITY:** While powders and pills can add fiber to your diet, getting your fiber from foods is generally better for your health. Fiber supplements do not provide the vitamins, minerals, and other beneficial nutrients that high-fiber foods do. In addition, fiber supplements don't give you the crunchy satisfaction and feeling of fullness that comes from eating fiber-rich foods. The bottom line is, it's best to try to satisfy your fiber needs with foods. Save fiber supplements for when you simply cannot make the recommended intake or if your doctor prescribes them.

**6. MYTH:** All dark breads and wheat products are a good source of fiber.

**REALITY:** Just because a label says "whole wheat" or "made with whole grains" does not mean a food is high in fiber. Many breads and cereals claim to be made from whole grains and yet contain very little fiber. Some brown breads are part whole wheat and part white flour with caramel coloring added to make them appear more wholesome. Read the ingredient label to be sure. Look for items made from 100 percent whole wheat—these will have the most fiber. Select breads with at least 3 grams of fiber per slice. For a list of recommended breads, see Appendix B on page 271.

**7. MYTH:** Eating high-fiber foods will make you feel bloated.

**REALITY:** People who typically eat a *low*-fiber diet may experience some initial minor bloating and abdominal cramps when they begin to eat large amounts of fiber. It is important to introduce fiber-rich foods slowly, which is why Step 1 limits your fiber intake to three servings of high-fiber carbohydrates, making it unlikely that you will eat too much fiber too quickly. For the few patients who do experience some initial discomfort, it goes away within a few days as their bodies become accustomed to eating fiber on a daily basis. In fact, practically *all* patients report *flatter* stomachs and *less bloat* after just two weeks on the F-Factor Diet.

**8. MYTH:** It is possible to eat too much fiber.

**REALITY:** Some health care experts believe that eating more than 80 grams of fiber per day may adversely affect vitamin and mineral absorption. While this is technically true, rarely does anyone eat nearly that amount of fiber. Most of us don't eat even the small amount we need (26–38 grams/day). Don't let the fear of becoming nutrient deficient stop you from boosting your fiber intake. The benefits of fiber far outweigh the remote possibility that you will eat quantities large enough to pose any problem. Keep track in your daily journal, and follow the guidelines for the three steps on the F-Factor Diet.

**9. MYTH:** "If I'm not constipated, I don't need to worry about fiber."

**REALITY:** This is certainly false! Just because you are regular does not mean you are getting enough fiber. Fiber does much more than relieve occasional constipation. Not only does a high-fiber diet help keep your digestive system healthy, it may reduce the risk factors for cardiovascular disease, adult-onset diabetes, and certain forms of cancer. A high-fiber diet is also the healthiest way to lose weight and keep it off.

10. MYTH: Fiber-rich foods are found only in health food stores, not my local supermarket.
REALITY: Your local supermarket is filled with high-fiber foods. Aside from the fresh fruits and vegetables, the shelves are stocked with high-fiber foods including breads, cold and hot cereals, breakfast bars, cookies, popcorn, whole-wheat pretzels, brown rice, whole-wheat pasta, crackers, nuts, and much more. F-Factor's line of high-fiber products are available for purchase at www.FFactor .com and other online retailers. As fiber awareness grows, you can expect to see even more high-fiber products introduced to the marketplace in the months to come.

# THE PROGRAM:
# THE F-FACTOR DIET

CHAPTER

## 6

# STEP 1:
# JUMP-START YOUR WEIGHT LOSS

*Though no one can go back and make a brand-new start, anyone
can start from now and make a brand-new ending.*
—CARL BARD

THE PURPOSE of Step 1 is to boost your weight loss immediately. Unlike other diets that prohibit one food group or another, the F-Factor Diet includes all food groups from day one. You will eat protein, fat, *and* even carbohydrates—wisely and effectively.

During Step 1 you are encouraged to eat three servings of carbohydrate a day: a serving of a high-fiber cereal, a serving of fresh fruit (over 25 to choose from), and up to 8 high-fiber crackers. In addition, you get to consume substantial quantities of protein from the very lean and lean protein lists and as many vegetables from the nonstarchy vegetable list as you would like. You may also include some healthy fat, such as a handful of nuts for a snack, or a few slices of avocado for your salad. Keeping daily journals—a sample journal page is included near the end of this chapter—will guide you in your effort to meet your goals of at least 35 grams fiber and less than 35 grams *net carbohydrate* a day.

Although Step 1 is the most restrictive step of the F-Factor Diet, its guidelines deliver three great initial benefits:

1. You'll become instantly aware of just how dependent on carbohydrates your current dietary habits are. By eliminating—just for these two weeks—all but the three specific allowable carbohydrates mentioned above, you'll not only become acutely aware of what a carbohydrate is and is not, you'll also become mindful of how many carbohydrates you've actually been eating before starting this program. Do you typically eat a sandwich and bag of chips for lunch? Is dinner often a bowl of pasta? None of those foods are allowed on Step 1, and your awareness of your eating habits is the first necessary step toward changing your weight permanently.

2. Your gastrointestinal tract needs time to adjust to an increase in fiber consumption. With fiber, initially there is such a thing as "too much of a good thing." Adding too much fiber too quickly may lead to discomfort. Since most Americans eat less than half of the recommended fiber in the F-Factor Diet, the healthiest way to add fiber is to do it slowly. Step 1 introduces three servings of high-fiber carbohydrates to your diet, ensuring that you incorporate fiber into your diet, but not so much as to cause any discomfort. After two weeks on Step 1, your body will have become accustomed to that amount of fiber, and you will be ready to add even more fiber in Step 2.

3. You will experience immediate weight loss—a 4- to 6-pound weight loss in this initial two-week Step 1 will motivate you to carry on with the program. Keep in mind that although Step 1 is the most challenging part, it provides the incentive you need to continue successfully. After Step 1, it only gets easier.

The one thing you *won't* feel during these initial two weeks is hungry. On Step 1, you'll be *required* to eat three full meals and one snack a day—no skipping allowed. The reason for not skipping meals is that when you go too many hours without eating your body thinks you're fasting, causing the body to store fat rather than burn it, in case there's a food shortage developing. In addition, allowing too many hours between meals causes fatigue and low blood sugar, which leads to overeating at the next meal. By eating breakfast, lunch, a snack, and dinner, you are guaranteed to feel full, have energy, and keep your metabolism working efficiently. Losing weight becomes effortless.

## Your Shopping List

High-fiber crackers (such as GG Bran Crispbreads, which have 6 grams of carbohydrate and 4 grams of fiber each)

Cereal: Fiber One, All-Bran, Original or All-Bran Bran Buds, Nature's Path SmartBran

Fruits and vegetables

Cheese: 1% cottage cheese, nonfat or low-fat cheese slices (Kraft, Alpine Lace), Laughing Cow Light, string cheese

Yogurt: 0% fat plain Greek or Icelandic yogurt, or 0% fat plain quark

Meat and meat substitutes:

- eggs, Egg Beaters
- tuna fish canned in water
- lean cold cuts: turkey, chicken, ham, and roast beef
- meats (if you cook): chicken breast, lean cuts of beef, pork, lamb, veal, and fish
- unsweetened almond milk

Frozen treats: Tofutti Chocolate Fudge Treats, sugar-free ice pops, Arctic Zero Creamy Pints

Sugar-free Jell-O

F-Factor Fiber/Protein products

## Limit Carbohydrates

For the next two weeks, you'll follow Step 1 of the F-Factor Diet. During this time, you will eat a limited amount of carbohydrates. The carbohydrates allowed are:

1. Fiber One, All-Bran Original or Nature's Path SmartBran (½ cup per day), or All-Bran Bran Buds (⅓ cup per day)
2. High-fiber crackers, such as GG Bran Crispbreads (up to 8 per day)
3. 1 serving of fruit per day

Limiting your net carbohydrate intake to less than 35 grams per day will result in optimum weight loss and help teach you how easy it is to overeat carbohydrates, as well as which foods contain carbohydrates (starch, fruit, milk, and yogurt). After two weeks, you will begin Step 2.

Step 2 adds 3 more servings of carbohydrate into your daily eating plan.

## Add Protein

To make up for the overall cut in carbs, the F-Factor Diet permits ample amounts of protein. Each meal offers guidelines to meeting your protein needs:

- breakfast: 2–3 ounces of protein for women, 4–6 ounces for men
- lunch: 3–4 ounces of protein for women, 4–6 ounces for men
- snack: 2–4 ounces of protein for women, 4 ounces for men
- dinner: 3–4 ounces of protein for women, 4–6 ounces for men

Average protein intake on the F-Factor Diet is 10 to 22 ounces a day. An ounce of protein has 7 grams of protein, therefore, intake on the F-Factor Diet ranges from 70 to 154 grams per day. Unlike many high-protein diets that allow you to eat high-fat meats and cheeses, the F-Factor Diet recommends proteins from the very lean and lean protein lists, keeping unhealthy saturated fat to a minimum. Lean meats, poultry, fish, seafood, and eggs are all good sources of lean protein. Lean dairy products such as low-fat cheeses are nutritious and not fattening and provide calcium for healthy bones. Every meal and snack on the F-Factor Diet should be a combination of fiber and protein. Filling up on lean protein and fiber is the secret to losing weight without feeling hungry. Remember:

Fiber and protein at every meal
Makes losing weight no big deal!

There is a space on the journal page where you are to fill in what protein you ate. This serves as a reminder that you should have some protein, along with high-fiber carbohydrates, at every meal: breakfast, lunch, snack, and dinner.

## How Much Protein Do I Need?

The typical American diet provides plenty of protein—more than twice the RDA in most instances. The amount of protein needed per day differs from person to person because it is based on how much you weigh. For healthy adults, the recommended dietary allowance (RDA) for protein is 0.8 grams of protein per kilogram of body weight. For a 150-pound person, that would be about 55 grams of protein per day. Here's how you calculate your own protein needs: divide your weight in pounds by 2.2, multiply that number by 0.8, and the remaining number is how many grams of protein you should aim to eat per day.

All protein you eat should be chosen from the very lean and lean lists from the exchange lists in Chapter 3. Please rely on the exchange lists to monitor carbohydrates and fiber, and do not forget to keep a journal. Documenting what you eat every day for the next two weeks is important.

## Do I Really Have to Keep a Journal?

Recording what you eat in a journal is one of the best ways to keep you accountable for everything you eat. It's like the saying, "If a tree falls in the forest and no one hears it, does it make a sound?" The same can apply to eating. If you grabbed a handful of M&M's but didn't acknowledge it by writing it down, then do the calories count? The answer is: of course. But surprisingly, many people do not account for a handful of chips or a bite of dessert, when in reality all these calories can add up.

In addition, journaling can help you evaluate the nutritional composition of your diet. A quick look at your journals may reveal that you don't eat enough fruits or vegetables, or that you eat too much fat. Keeping a journal can also expose patterns of eating that you weren't aware of. Do you turn to food when you feel sad or angry? Do you tend to consume most of your calories in the evening rather than spread them out during the day? Becoming aware of your diet patterns and eating behaviors is the first step toward change.

The journals in this book are tools that I created to ensure your success on the F-Factor Diet. Steps 1, 2, and 3 each have a corresponding journal that outlines the goals for fiber and total carbohydrate intake. The F-Factor App provides similar journaling capability as well. The journals are your safety net—they catch you from falling off the program. By recording everything you ate that day, along with the carbohydrate and fiber contents, you'll know on a daily basis whether you're eating the target amount of fiber and carbohydrates that will lead to weight loss. My patients report that the journals are an essential tool to help them follow and succeed on the program.

## How to Use the Journal

A blank journal form accompanies each step of the F-Factor Diet. For each step, the fiber goal remains at least 35 grams per day, while the net carbohydrate goal changes. While you are on Step 1, the net carbohydrate goal is 35 grams or less. On Step 2, your goal will be 75 grams, and on Step 3, you'll consume an average of less than 125 grams net carbohydrate per day. As you progress on the program, your net carbohydrate allowance increases.

Before starting Step 1, you will need to either download the F-Factor App or make 14 copies of the Step 1 journal (found on page 91)—one for each day of your first two weeks. You must keep your journal every day for a total of 14 days. Every day, after each meal, you will record what you ate. Next to foods that contain carbohydrate, write in their carbohydrate and fiber content.

Use the appendix, exchange lists, and food labels to fill in the correct numbers.

Remember, the only food groups considered carbohydrates on the F-Factor Diet are the starch, fruit/juice, milk/yogurt groups. Nonstarchy vegetables are considered to have no carbohydrates, and meat and meat substitutes and fat also have no carbohydrate.

Although nonstarchy vegetables are not counted as carbohydrates, I still want you to benefit from their fiber content. So when you eat vegetables, enter in a zero for carbohydrate, and fill in their fiber using the nonstarchy vegetable exchange list as a reference.

Let's take a look at a sample of a Step 1 journal.

| Date   Monday, June 11 | Carb | Fiber |
|---|---|---|
| **BREAKFAST** | | |
| 1 (6 oz) cup plain non-fat Greek yogurt | 0 | 0 |
| 1/3 cup All-Bran Bran Buds | 24 | 13 |
| 3/4 cup blueberries | 15 | 5 |
| | | |
| **LUNCH** | | |
| Artichoke salad with Parmesan cheese | 0 | 6 |
| Tuna tartare | 0 | 0 |
| **SNACK** | | |
| 4 F-Factor "Pizzas" | 24 | 16 |
| **DINNER/SUPPER** | | |
| Shrimp cocktail with 2 tbsp. cocktail sauce | 0 | 0 |
| 6 oz. grilled filet mignon | 0 | 0 |
| ½ cup sautéed mushrooms | 0 | 2 |
| ½ cup grilled asparagus | 0 | 2 |
| 1 vodka martini | 0 | 0 |
| **SNACK/DESSERT** | | |
| 1 Tofutti Chocolate Fudge Treats pop | 6 | 0 |
| | | |
| | 69 g | 44 g |
| | A | B = >35 g |

**A – B = C**

69 g – 44 g = 25 g     (25 g)

ingested carb    fiber

<35 g net carb/day

## Journal Tips

On Step 1, the only carbohydrates allowed are Fiber One, All-Bran Original, All-Bran Bran Buds, or Nature's Path SmartBran cereal; high-fiber crackers; and 1 serving of fruit. The cereals have 20–27 grams of carbohydrate and 10–14 grams of fiber (look at the nutrition facts label for each cereal for the exact amount). The recommended high-fiber cracker is the GG Bran Crispbread, which has 6 grams of carbohydrate and 4 grams of fiber each. Finally, fruit has 15 grams of carbohydrate per serving (exchange list standard). Use the exchange lists to determine the amount of fiber in the specific fruit you choose.

When you document the vegetables you eat in your journal, allot vegetables a zero for grams of carbohydrate. Although vegetables contain some carbohydrate, remember that on the F-Factor Diet they are considered a carbohydrate-free food. But do give yourself the benefit of the fiber they contain. Use the nonstarchy vegetables exchange lists to look up the fiber content. Meat and meat substitutes contain zero carbohydrate and zero fiber. Fats (except avocado and nuts) also are carbohydrate- and fiber-free, so leave them blank.

*Summary for Journaling on Step 1*

| FOOD | CARBOHYDRATE | FIBER |
|---|---|---|
| Cereal | | |
|     Nature's Path SmartBran | 24 g | 13 g |
|     Fiber One | 25 g | 14 g |
|     All-Bran Bran Buds | 24 g | 13 g |
|     All-Bran Original | 23 g | 10 g |
| GG Bran Crispbread (per cracker) | 6 g | 4 g |
| Fruit | 15 g | Look up on Exchange List in Chap. 3 |
| Vegetables | 0 g | Look up on Exchange List in Chap. 3 |
| Proteins | 0 g | 0 g |
| Fats | 0 g | Look up on Exchange List in Chap. 3 |
| 0% fat Greek yogurt | 0 g | 0 g |
| 0–1% fat cottage cheese | 0 g | 0 g |

## STEP 1 JOURNAL

| Date | | Carb | Fiber |
|---|---|---|---|
| **BREAKFAST** | | | |
| | | | |
| | | | |
| | | | |
| | | | |
| **LUNCH** | | | |
| | | | |
| | | | |
| | | | |
| | | | |
| | | | |
| **SNACK** | | | |
| | | | |
| | | | |
| **DINNER/SUPPER** | | | |
| | | | |
| | | | |
| | | | |
| | | | |
| | | | |
| **SNACK/DESSERT** | | | |
| | | | |
| | | | |

$$A \quad - \quad B \quad = \quad C$$
$$g \quad - \quad g \quad = \quad g$$

ingested carb        fiber

( )  **<35 g net carb/day**

| g | g |
|---|---|
| A | B = >35 g |

After entering all the carbohydrate and fiber contents, add them up.

1. Add up all the carbohydrates and put the sum on the total line above the letter A. This is your total number of ingested carbohydrate. On the sample journal, you'll see the total is 69 grams.
2. Next, add up the fiber and place the sum on the total line above the letter B. On the sample, the total for fiber is 44 grams.
3. Finally, subtract the total fiber (B) from the total digestible carbohydrate (A) to get your net carbohydrate intake, which is 25 grams.

**A** (total ingested carbohydrate) − **B** (fiber) = **C** (net digestible carbohydrate)

Since fiber is the indigestible portion of carbohydrate, you subtract the fiber from the total ingested carbohydrate to figure out how much carbohydrate actually gets digested. The goal on Step 1 is to keep the net digestible carbohydrate below 35 grams a day. From the example, you can see how much food you can eat throughout the day and still reach your goals for fiber and net carbohydrate.

When it comes to losing weight for the long term, counting calories and restrictive meals do not work. Flexible dieting, on the other hand, is linked to slimmer figures, fewer binges, and less depression and anxiety.

Try to remain conscious of what you are eating throughout the day, and record your meals in a journal. So before you order dinner, review what you have eaten up to that point and adjust your choices accordingly.

## No Skipping Meals or Snacks

Skipping meals does not help weight loss or dieting!

Many people mistakenly believe that by skipping meals, they will save on calories, and lose more weight. Surprisingly, skipping meals may inhibit weight loss and even lead to weight gain over time. When your body is deprived of food for many hours between meals, it starts conserving fuel and burning fewer calories to protect itself from starving. Your metabolism slows down, therefore inhibiting weight loss despite reduced caloric intake. In addition, skipping meals causes sugar levels to begin to drop. Low blood sugar can produce sudden hunger pangs, which can trigger bingeing and food cravings. Blood sugar levels begin to drop within four hours of eating, which is why I recommend eating breakfast no later than an hour after rising, and then following that with lunch, a snack, and dinner at four- to five-hour intervals. For example:

8:00 A.M. breakfast
12:00–1:00 P.M. lunch
4:00–5:00 P.M. afternoon snack
6:00–8:00 P.M. dinner

Regular, frequent meals and snacks rather than two or three big meals are the best bet for maintaining a constant energy supply and avoiding fatigue.

Of all the meals that people choose to skip, breakfast is the most common. Some people say they simply aren't hungry when they wake up while others claim that lack of time in the morning is the reason. Whatever the excuse, skipping breakfast is one of the worst things you can do if you are trying to lose weight. Breakfast is not only essential for your physical and mental health but recent research shows that eating breakfast can actually help you shed pounds. A 1992 study at Vanderbilt University found that women who changed their diet to include breakfast lost 28 percent more weight over a 12-week period than women who skipped their morning repast. In addition, a full 78 percent of the 3,000 people enrolled in the National Weight Loss Registry, an ongoing tally of adults who have lost at least 30 pounds and kept it off for more than a year, describe themselves as breakfast eaters.

## Diet Secrets of Breakfast Foods

How can eating breakfast help you manage your weight? The answer lies in the nutritional value of one of the most common breakfast foods: cereal. High-fiber cereals provide you with energy while making you feel full and curbing midmorning cravings. In fact, a recent national survey of consumer eating trends found that people who eat cereal weigh an average of 8 pounds less than those who don't. Not only do high-fiber cereals contain fewer calories than most breakfast foods, the fiber content helps to keep you full all morning long.

To dramatically reduce the risk of gaining weight, eat breakfast before you leave your home in the morning. A University of Massachusetts study of 499 people found that frequently eating breakfast away from home doubles the risk of becoming obese, probably because of the types of food and the portion sizes served in restaurants.

## Comparison of Breakfast Foods and Their Dietary Consequences

AT HOME:
bowl of All-Bran Bran Buds with ¾ cup blueberries and 1 cup of skim milk: 242 calories, 18 grams fiber

AWAY FROM HOME:
Dunkin' Donuts bagel with cream cheese: 430 calories, 4 grams fiber
Dunkin' Donuts glazed cake doughnut: 260 calories, 1 gram fiber
Dunkin' Donuts blueberry muffin: 460 calories, 2 grams fiber
McDonald's bacon, egg, and cheese biscuit: 450 calories, 3 grams fiber
McDonald's hotcakes and sausage: 790 calories, 2 grams fiber

You say making breakfast takes too much time? You can assemble a bowl of cereal with berries and milk in the same time it takes to toast a Pop Tart.

Planning and shopping for several weeks ahead will supply your kitchen with foods you will want to choose. If your kitchen is stocked with the foods you want, you won't be as tempted to run out and grab breakfast on your way to work. And you'll have a good F-Factor diet snack ready to tote to work with you or to enjoy the moment you get home.

# Foods Permitted on Step 1

On Step 1 you are permitted three specific carbohydrates:

1. ½ cup All-Bran Original, Fiber One Original, or Nature's Path SmartBran or ⅓ cup All-Bran Bran Buds cereal
2. High-fiber crackers, such as GG Bran Crispbreads (up to 8 a day)
3. 1 serving of fruit (look at the fruit exchange list for the correct portion size of your fruit choice)

In addition, you can eat as many nonstarchy vegetables as you like, and 2 to 6 ounces of lean or very lean meat or meat substitute (look at exchange lists) per meal (breakfast, lunch, snack, and dinner).

## VEGETABLES

artichoke

asparagus

beans (green, wax)

bean sprouts

beets

broccoli

Brussels sprouts

cabbage

carrots

cauliflower

celery

cucumber

eggplant

green onions or scallions

greens (collard, kale,
    mustard, turnip)

kohlrabi

leeks

mixed vegetables (without corn, peas)

mushrooms

okra

onions

pea pods

peppers

radishes

salad greens

spinach

summer squash

tomato

tomato sauce

tomato/vegetable juice

turnips

water chestnuts

watercress

zucchini

## VERY LEAN AND LEAN PROTEINS:

POULTRY

Cornish hen

turkey bacon

chicken/turkey lean sausage

chicken/turkey, no skin

BEEF (USDA SELECT OR CHOICE GRADE CUTS
    TRIMMED OF FAT)

round

sirloin

flank steak

tenderloin

roast (rib, chuck, rump)

steak (T-bone, porterhouse, cubed)

ground round

PORK

ham (canned, cured, or boiled)

Canadian bacon

tenderloin

center loin chop

LAMB

roast

chop

leg

VEAL

chop

cutlet (no breading)

GAME
duck or pheasant (skinless)
venison
buffalo
ostrich
goose (skinless)

FISH
catfish
cod
flounder
haddock
halibut
herring (uncreamed or smoked)
lox
oysters
salmon (fresh or canned)
sardines
sole
snapper
trout
tuna fish (fresh or canned in water)

SHELLFISH
clams
crab
lobster
scallops
shrimp
squid

CHEESE
fat-free or low-fat cottage cheese
fat-free or low-fat ricotta

fat-free or low-fat cheese (sliced, shredded)
Parmesan
feta and part-skim mozzarella (3 g fat or less per oz)

OTHER
fat-free or low-fat processed sandwich meats (turkey, ham, roast beef)
egg whites
egg substitute
whole eggs (no more than 3 a week)
fat-free or low-fat hot dogs
lite tofu
0% fat plain Greek or Icelandic yogurt

NUTS
almonds, 15
cashews, 15
PB2, 2 tbsp.
peanut butter, 2 tbsp.
peanuts, 20
pecan halves, 15

## FATS

avocado
low-fat mayonnaise
low-fat cream cheese
low-fat salad dressing
nonstick cooking spray
oils: canola, olive
olives

## SWEET/DESSERTS

Tofutti Chocolate Fudge Treats
sugar-free Popsicles
sugar-free jelly (2 teaspoons)
sugar-free gelatin with 1 tbsp.
    nonfat whipped topping
diet hot cocoa
Arctic Zero Creamy Pints

## CONDIMENTS

ketchup (1 tbsp.)
horseradish
lemon juice
lime juice
mustard
pickle relish (1 tbsp.)
pickles, dill
salsa
soy sauce, low-sodium
taco sauce
vinegar

## SEASONINGS

flavoring extracts
garlic
herbs, fresh or dried
pimento
spices
Tabasco or hot
    pepper sauce
Worcestershire sauce

## DRINKS

wine and spirits
carbonated or mineral water
club soda, diet tonic water
coffee
diet soft drinks, sugar-free
drink mixes, sugar-free
unsweetened tea
unsweetened almond milk

## Foods to Avoid on Step 1

**Starches:** Avoid all starchy food during Step 1, including all types of breads, cereals and grains, beans, peas, lentils, pasta, rice, pastries, crackers, snack foods, and baked goods.

**Starchy Vegetables and Legumes:** barley, beans, corn, peas, sweet potatoes, white potatoes, and yams

**Fruit:** You are allowed 1 serving of fresh fruit. *No fruit juice.*

**Milk/Yogurt:** Avoid all dairy foods during Step 1 including ice cream, milk, soy milk, and yogurt (except cheese, which is a protein). *The allowed exceptions:* 0% fat plain Greek or Icelandic yogurt and 0% fat plain quark.

**Medium-fat and High-fat Meats:**

- beef: brisket, liver, rib steaks, other fatty cuts
- poultry: all dark meat with skin: chicken wings, thighs and legs with skin, turkey wings, thighs and legs, duck, goose, fried chicken
- pork: spareribs, ground pork, pork sausage, shoulder and cutlet
- veal: breast
- cheese: Brie, Edam, all full-fat cheeses including Swiss and cheddar
- other: bacon, hot dogs, salami, bologna

---

## Step 1 Guidelines

**BREAKFAST**

Choose 1 from the options below. Option to pair with additional side.

### High-Fiber Cereal and Lean Protein:

½ cup All-Bran Original, Fiber One Original or Nature's Path SmartBran, or ⅓ cup All-Bran Bran Buds cereal with either:

- 1 cup 1–2% cottage cheese
- 6 ounces 0% fat plain Greek or Icelandic yogurt
- 1 cup unsweetened almond milk

### High-Fiber Crackers and Lean Protein:

Four high-fiber crackers, such as GG Bran crispbreads with any protein from the very lean or lean meat and meat substitutes list in Chapter 3. Examples include, but are not limited to:

- 2–4 egg whites, Egg Beaters or egg and egg white combination (1 egg yolk with 2 egg whites)
  - ➤ *Omelets/eggs can be made with your favorite vegetables and nonfat or low-fat cheese*
- ½ cup–1 cup 1–2% cottage cheese
- 2–4 ounces smoked salmon with 2 tbsp low-fat cream cheese

**Fiber and Protein on-the-Go:**
- High fiber/high protein smoothie or shake (see recipe on page 182 for example)
- F-Factor Fiber/Protein Bar

**Optional Sides:**
- 2 ounces turkey bacon, Canadian bacon, low-fat sausage, smoked salmon, or any lean or very lean protein
- serving of fruit
- nonstarchy vegetables

## LUNCH

Choose 1 from each category:

**Fiber:**
- Garden salad with oil and vinegar (no more than 2 tsp oil), light dressing, or squeeze of fresh lemon
- 1–2 cups fresh vegetables (crudités, salad, etc.)
- 1 cup gazpacho, vegetable soup, miso soup, or consommé with vegetables and chicken (no rice, pasta, potatoes, beans, or cream)

**Protein:**
3–6 ounces of any protein from the very lean or lean meat and meat substitutes list in Chapter 3. Examples include, but are not limited to:

- Tuna salad, chicken salad, or crab salad (prepared with nonfat mayonnaise)
- Tuna, salmon, crab meat, shrimp, or lobster
- Lunch meat: sliced turkey, lean ham, roast beef
- Poultry (no skin), lean beef
- Cottage cheese, part-skim mozzarella cheese
- Lite tofu

## SNACK

Choose 1:
- Four high-fiber crackers with protein from the very lean or lean meat and meat substitutes list in Chapter 3. Examples include, but are not limited to:

- ➤ ¼ cup cottage cheese and 1 Tbsp. sugar-free jelly
- ➤ 1–2 Tbsp. PB2 powdered peanut butter
- ➤ 2–4 ounces sliced turkey, roast beef, or low-fat cheese
- ➤ 2 hard-boiled eggs
- ➤ 4 ounces low fat tuna, chicken, or egg salad
- ➤ 2 Laughing Cow Light cheese wedges
- ➤ "Pizzas" made with 1% cottage cheese or part-skim mozzarella and sauce
- ¼ cup dried fruit mixed with ¼ cup nuts (peanuts, pecans, almonds, and/or pistachios)
- 1 mozzarella string cheese with 1 piece of fruit (if you have not had your serving of fruit for the day)
- 1 cup raw vegetables with ½ cup dip (made from blending onion or vegetable soup mix with 0% fat plain Greek yogurt)
- F-Factor Fiber/Protein Bar or high fiber/high protein shake

## DINNER

Choose 1 from each course/category:

### APPETIZERS/SIDES:

- Salad with low-fat or nonfat dressing
- Soup (broth-based, made without cream, potatoes, pasta, rice, or beans)

### VEGETABLES:

- Any vegetables (from the nonstarchy vegetables list) steamed, sautéed, or grilled (prepared with minimum oil)

### MAIN COURSE:

4–6 ounces of any protein from the very lean or lean lists in Chapter 3. Examples include, but are not limited to:

- Beef: lean cuts such as sirloin, tenderloin, flank steak, ground round, and top round
- Poultry: chicken or turkey (no skin), Cornish hen (no skin), duck (well drained of fat, no skin), ground chicken, or turkey breast (99% lean)
- Seafood: all types of fish and shellfish (broiled, grilled, steamed, poached—not fried)

- Pork: boiled ham, Canadian bacon, tenderloin, center loin chop
- Veal: chop, leg cutlet, top round
- Cheese (fat-free or low-fat): American, cheddar, 1% fat cottage cheese, fat-free or low-fat cream cheese, feta, mozzarella, Parmesan, provolone, and ricotta

**DESSERT (OPTIONAL):**
- Sugar-free Jell-O
- 1 Tofutti Chocolate Fudge Treat
- ½ cup Arctic Zero Creamy Pints
- sugar-free ice pop
- diet hot chocolate
- 1 small serving of fruit (*if you haven't already used your 1 serving of fruit earlier in the day*)

# A Sample Menu Plan and Corresponding Journal for Step 1

**BREAKFAST**

1 cup mixed berries
scrambled eggs with fresh herbs and mushrooms
turkey bacon, 2 slices
4 GG Bran Crispbreads

**LUNCH**

large chopped vegetable salad (lettuce, cucumber, carrot, broccoli, tomato) with grilled chicken and 2 tbsp. mustard vinaigrette
unsweetened iced tea

**MIDAFTERNOON SNACK**

4 GG Bran Crispbreads with 2 oz turkey breast and mustard

**DINNER**

kale salad with 2 tbsp. vinaigrette
6 oz grilled branzino

THE F-FACTOR DIET

| Date Monday, June 11 | Carb | Fiber |
|---|---|---|
| **BREAKFAST** | | |
| 1 cup mixed berries | 15 | 5 |
| Scrambled eggs with fresh herbs and mushrooms | 0 | 2 |
| Turkey bacon, 2 slices | 0 | 0 |
| 4 GG Bran Crispbreads | 24 | 16 |
| **LUNCH** | | |
| Chopped vegetable salad | 0 | 5 |
| grilled chicken | 0 | 0 |
| 2 tbsp mustard vinaigrette | 0 | 0 |
| unsweetened iced tea | 0 | 0 |
| | | |
| **SNACK** | | |
| 4 GG Bran Crispbreads | 24 | 16 |
| Turkey breast (with mustard) | 0 | 0 |
| **DINNER/SUPPER** | | |
| Kale salad | 0 | 2 |
| Grilled branzino | 0 | 0 |
| 1 cup sautéed broccoli | 0 | 4 |
| 2 glasses white wine | 4 | 0 |
| | | |
| **SNACK/DESSERT** | | |
| 1/2 cup Chocolate Peanut Butter Arctic Zero | 7 | 2 |

|  |  |  |  | Carb | Fiber |
|---|---|---|---|---|---|
| **A** | **– B** | **= C** | | 74 g | 52 g |
| 74 g | – 52 g | = 22 g | **(22)** | | |
| ingested carb | fiber | | | **A** | **B >35 g** |

<35 g net carb/day

1 cup sautéed broccoli

2 glasses white wine

## DESSERT

½ cup Chocolate Peanut Butter Arctic Zero

## DON'T FORGET (ALL PHASES)

1. Drink at least 8 glasses of water or decaf beverages per day (club soda, unsweetened flavored seltzers, decaf tea or coffee, decaf, sugar-free sodas).
2. Take a daily multivitamin and mineral supplement.
3. Take a daily calcium supplement (500 mg for men of all ages and women under 50, 1,000 mg for women over 50).

## Frequently Asked Questions on Step 1

QUESTION: How do I know if my cracker qualifies as a high-fiber cracker?

ANSWER: On Step 1, you can use any cracker that fits the following parameters: each cracker should be less than 30 calories with at least 4 grams of fiber and no more than 2 net carbs. To calculate the net carbs, you subtract the dietary fiber from the total carbohydrate. A look at the GG Bran Crispbread nutrition label reveals that each cracker contains 6 grams of carbohydrate and 4 grams of fiber.

$$6 \text{ g carbohydrate} - 4 \text{ g fiber} = 2 \text{ g net carbs}$$

In essence, these crackers pass through your digestive tract without increasing your serum glucose levels. High-fiber crackers like the GG Bran Crispbreads are basically indigestible fiber crackers. When cutting back on carbohydrates, these crackers offer you the opportunity to eat something crunchy and filling without digesting a high level of carbohydrates. To make them even tastier, and to get the combination of fiber and protein, you can top them with a lean protein of your choice. For example, top them with tuna salad, sliced turkey breast, or spread on a layer of peanut butter.

QUESTION: We learned earlier that milk and yogurt are carbohydrates. Since Step 1 allows for only three carbohydrates (a high-fiber cereal, high-fiber crackers, and 1 serving of fruit), why am I allowed to eat 0% fat Greek or Icelandic yogurt and 0% fat plain quark?

ANSWER: In Chapter 3, you learned that milk and yogurt contain 15 grams of carbohydrate, the same amount of carbohydrate as a serving of starch or fruit. So why do I make the exception for 0% fat plain Greek or Icelandic yogurt and 0% fat plain quark? The answer lies in their nutritional content.

Both fat-free Greek and Icelandic yogurt, as well as fat-free plain quark, have 6 grams of carbohydrate and 0 grams fiber.

None of these products have close to 15 grams of carbohydrate, which would place them solidly in the carbohydrate group. The non-carbohydrate groups (nonstarchy vegetables, meat and meat substitutes, and fat) have 0 grams of carbohydrate. Therefore, 0% fat plain Greek yogurt, 0% fat plain Icelandic yogurt, and 0% fat plain quark fall in between the two groups. Since Step 1 is so limited, I have included these foods in this part of the program because they are both sources of protein and calcium, are low in carbohydrates, and provide additional eating variety. For those of you who don't like cottage cheese, these yogurts are a delicious and nutritional alternative when combining them with your fiber cereal, especially in the absence of drinking milk.

QUESTION: Why should I take a multivitamin?

ANSWER: A multivitamin provides nutrients to supplement a healthy (or unhealthy) diet. Of course it's possible—and preferable—to get your nutrients from a healthy, balanced diet. But surveys show that many Americans fall short in a variety of key vitamins and minerals. Moreover, many studies suggest that people who take multivitamin/mineral pills have a lower risk of several diseases, including colon cancer and possibly cardiovascular disease, and may have a better immune response.

Think of a multivitamin as health insurance. While most days you may eat 100 percent of the RDA for vitamins and nutrients, some days you may not. Since Step 1 limits the amounts of fresh fruit and whole grains in your diet, by taking a multivitamin you ensure that despite a few temporary diet shortcomings, you will be getting enough of the recommended daily vitamins.

Keep in mind that multivitamins are not magic bullets. You should not rely on them for your vitamin and mineral needs. Nothing can replace a healthy, balanced diet. Foods—particularly fruits, vegetables, and whole grains—provide fiber as well as countless beneficial phytochemicals not found in any pill.

QUESTION: Is it really important that I drink 8 glasses of water a day?

ANSWER: Water plays a key role in nearly every bodily function, including digestion, circulation, and regulating body temperature. In addition, water fills you up so you tend to eat less. When you don't drink enough fluids your body gets dehydrated and you may feel weak, shaky, or tired. Often people confuse these symptoms with hunger so they grab something to eat. They take in unnecessary calories, when in reality they just needed to drink some fluids.

While drinking 8 glasses of water is an important part of most diets, it is *essential* to feeling your best on the F-Factor Diet. When fiber combines with water, it forms a soft gel, which leads to firm stools and allows for easy defecation. On the other hand, if you eat a lot of fiber and don't compensate by drinking more water, it can lead to the opposite effect—constipation. Think about what would happen if you took dry newspaper and shoved it down your sink drain. Without water to soften it, the paper would get lodged in the pipes. But add enough water, the newspaper softens and passes though the pipes with ease.

If you find water too "boring," you can boost the flavor by adding fresh lemon or Crystal Light powders. Crystal Light now comes in On-the-Go packets, individual packets that you add to a half-liter water bottle, or 2 cups of water. The packets are sugar-free, contain 0 carbohydrate and only 10 calories. My favorite flavor is Sunrise—it tastes like orange juice and provides 100 percent of the daily value for vitamin C without all the fructose in regular orange juice.

Drink diet soda and carbonated beverages in moderation. Carbonated beverages frequently contain added phosphorus in the form of phosphates, which have been shown to increase loss of calcium in the urine.[18] Significant

18. "Carbonated Beverages and Bone Fractures in Adolescent Girls," *American Family Physician*, 8–94. Also see C. Northrup, *Women's Bodies, Women's Wisdom* (New York: Bantam, 2002), 538.

lack of calcium may lead to bone loss and an increased risk for osteoporosis. While this issue is very controversial and remains unsettled, few think that drinking soda offers actual health benefits. Risks associated with soft drink consumption may be related more to associated behaviors—carbonated beverages often displace milk in the diet, eliminating a major source of bone-building calcium.

What is known for sure is that carbonated beverages can leave you feeling bloated. In addition, some studies suggest that drinking diet soft drinks stimulates appetite. What is the point of drinking a zero-calorie beverage if it leads you to consume more calories late in the day? Treat soda as a special treat and choose water as your staple beverage.

QUESTION: Are there other foods I can eat besides the examples given in the sample plan?

ANSWER: The sample plan is merely an outline of suggestions for meals on Step 1. Of course, there are many foods not on the sample plan that can be enjoyed on the F-Factor Diet. The key to remember is that every meal should be a combination of fiber and protein.

FIBER SOURCES:
- Fiber One, Nature's Path SmartBran, All-Bran Original and All-Bran Bran Buds
- High-fiber crackers, such as GG Bran Crispbreads
- A serving of fruit from the fruit list
- Vegetables from the nonstarchy vegetables list
- F-Factor Fiber/Protein products

PROTEIN SOURCES:
- Foods on the very lean and lean meat and meat substitute list
- 0% fat plain Greek or Icelandic yogurt, and 0% fat plain quark
- Nuts and nut spreads

As long as each meal consists of one fiber-rich food and one protein food, there are hundreds of combinations you can create to satisfy your appetite. Get inspired and see what works best for you.

# STEP 2: CONTINUED WEIGHT LOSS

*I do not think there is any other quality so essential to success of any kind as the quality of perseverance. It overcomes almost everything, even nature.*
—JOHN D. ROCKEFELLER

CONGRATULATIONS on completing Step 1!

The good news is that the hardest part is over. Reducing your carbohydrate intake for two full weeks is a challenge. But the rewards should certainly outweigh the changes you have made in your diet. After two weeks on Step 1, you can expect to have:

- lost a few pounds. By reducing your carbohydrate intake, you have lost both water weight (released from your glycogen stores) and stored body fat
- improved your metabolism
- experienced fewer mood swings and feelings of fatigue
- slept better
- felt less bloated
- had fewer cravings for carbohydrates

- understood more about which groups are considered carbohydrates (bagels, rice, pasta, bread, fruit, juice, milk, and yogurt) and which are not (meat, poultry, fish, eggs, cheese, and nonstarchy vegetables)

Step 2 adds 3 servings of carbohydrate to your current eating plan. You can combine all 3 servings of carbohydrates for 1 meal (for example, 1 cup of rice with dinner), or divide them into 3 meals (1 serving of carbohydrate at breakfast, lunch, and dinner). You decide!

## Serving Reminders:

1 serving = 15 g carbohydrate
2 servings = 30 g carbohydrate
3 servings = 45 g carbohydrate

In essence, you will be adding an additional 45 grams of carbohydrate to your Step 1 eating plan. Your goal for fiber remains the same: at least 35 grams per day but your goal for net carbohydrate intake on Step 2 has increased to 75 grams per day (up from 35 grams on Step 1).

## Adding in Carbohydrates

So which three carbohydrates are you going to add? The answer is completely up to you! If you love fruit, now is the time to add more into your diet. Or perhaps you are craving pasta—now you can have a cup. Step 2 gives you the freedom to choose the carbohydrates you want. The liberty to decide which foods to add to your diet is what personalizes this program for each individual and what makes this program work. While Step 1 is the most "dietlike" part of this program because of food limitations and boundaries, Step 2 begins the process of helping you create a healthy eating plan that fits in with your likes and lifestyle.

When choosing your 3 servings of carbohydrate to add, it is important to rely on the exchange lists in Chapter 3 for accurate portions. Typical portions of foods sold in restaurants, vending machines, and convenience stores exceed the standard exchanges many times over. You may think that adding

3 servings of carbohydrates sounds like a lot of food, but take a quick look at the exchange lists and you will see that 3 servings isn't nearly as much as you might think (or hope for!).

For example, when you dine on Chinese food, most entrées come with a cup of rice. You may think that would equal 1 serving. But a quick glance at the exchange lists reveals that a serving of rice is ⅓ cup. Therefore a cup of rice would actually use up all 3 daily servings!

Do you like raisins? A mere 2 *tablespoons* equals a serving.

Want milk in your cereal? One cup of milk equals 1 serving of carbohydrate.

You can see that the 3 servings add up quickly without contributing a lot of food.

## How Much of a Food Can I Eat? Learning to Read Food Labels

Learning to read food labels is essential for Step 2. Almost all packaged foods have a nutrition facts label that states nutritional value. Among other information, the nutrition facts label indicates the carbohydrate and fiber content of a serving. With this information, you can figure out how much of that food you are entitled to eat, while remaining within the parameters of Step 2 of the F-Factor Diet.

### How to Read Food Labels

The first step to reading the nutrition facts label is to look at how many servings a package contains. Your eye may naturally seek the calories first, or total carbohydrate or even fiber. It is important, though, to check the serving size first because the amounts of calories, carbohydrates, and fiber are all based on a single serving. If you eat a portion that equals 2 servings, multiply the calories and all the other amounts by 2.

Chips, candy bars, and soft drinks are among the many foods that have been jumbo-sized. Although they deceptively appear to be single servings, the nutrition facts label may reveal something altogether different. A candy bar looks like only one serving (who doesn't eat the entire bar?), but upon reading the label, you may be surprised that the nutrition facts state that the 1 bar consists of 2 servings. Therefore, however many calories or grams of carbohydrate a food label says, you may have to double or triple the amount if you plan on eating the whole thing.

The next step is to look at the carbohydrate and fiber contents. Subtract the amount of fiber from the carbohydrate to assess how much net (or digestible) carbohydrate is in a serving of that particular food. Keep in mind that a serving equals 15 grams, but you are entitled to add 45 grams to your day on Step 2. If a food contains 30 grams of digestible carbohydrate, then you have used up 2 of your 3 servings by eating that food.

Perhaps, for example, you decide you want to eat some Triscuits crackers. You grab the box and read the label:

**Nutrition Facts** Serving size: 6 crackers, Servings per container: About 9, Amount per serving: **Calories** 120, **Fat Cal.** 30, Total Fat NaNg (5%DV), Sat. Fat .5g (3%DV), **Cholesterol** 0mg (0%DV), **Sodium** 220 mg (7%DV), **Total Carb.** 20g (7%DV), Fiber 3g (12%DV), Sugars less than 1g, **Protein** 3g, Vitamin A (0% DV), Vitamin C (0%DV), Calcium (0%DV), Iron (8%DV). Percent Daily Values (DV) are based on a 2,000 calorie diet.

A serving contains 6 crackers, which provide you with 20 grams of total carbohydrate and 3 grams of fiber. When you subtract the fiber from the total carbohydrate, you are left with 17 grams of digestible carbohydrate. A serving of carbohydrate is 15 grams, so if you were to eat 6 Triscuits, you will have used up only 1 of your 3 additional servings of carbohydrate.

Perhaps you have plans to rent a movie and want to munch some popcorn. You grab a box of Orville Redenbacher's Smart Pop! microwave popcorn and read the label:

**Nutrition Facts** Serving Size: 3 Tbsp unpopped (makes about 7 cups popped), Servings Per Bag: about 2, Amount per serving: **Calories** 120, **Fat Cal.** 20, Total Fat 2 (3%V), Sat. Fat 0 (0%DV), Trans Fat 0, **Cholesterol** 0g (0%DV), **Sodium** 420mg (18%DV), **Total Carb**. 28g (9%DV), Fiber 7g (28%DV), Protein 4g, Iron 6%. (DV) are based on a 2,000 calorie diet.

If you subtract the fiber from the total carbohydrate, you are left with 21 grams of carbohydrate, or 1½ servings. But keep in mind that this is for half the bag. If you were to eat the entire bag, you would be eating 42 grams of digestible carbohydrate, which equals practically all 3 servings of your additional carbohydrates. You can eat the entire bag; just plan your day accordingly. Eat no other additional carbohydrates, and you can eat the whole bag, while maintaining the 45 grams of additional carbohydrate goal of Step 2.

Step 2 empowers you to eat almost any food in existence while remaining true to the program and continuing to lose weight. Sounds too good to be true? I assure you it's not. Let's say you are on Step 2 and are in the mood for Peanut M&M's. Can you eat them and still stick with Step 2? The answer is yes. Let's see how.

Here is the nutrition facts label for a bag of Peanut M&M's.

---

**Nutrition Facts**  Serving size: 1 pack, Amount per serving: **Calories** 240, **Fat Cal.** 90, Total Fat 10g (15%DV), Sat. Fat 6g (30%DV), Trans Fat 0g, **Cholesterol** 5mg (2%DV), **Sodium** 30mg (1%DV), **Total Carb.** 34g (11%DV), Fiber 1g (4%DV), Sugars 30g, **Protein** 2g, Vitamin A (0%DV), Vitamin C (0%DV), Calcium (4%DV), Iron (2%DV), Thiamine (2%DV), Riboflavin (4%DV), Niacin (8%DV). Percent Daily Values (DV) are based on a 2,000 calorie diet.

---

The serving size equals the entire package, so you know that the nutrition information applies to eating 1 bag. The total carbohydrate is 34 grams. Subtract the 1 gram of fiber from that. You are left with 33 grams of digestible carbohydrate, which is a little over 2 of your 3 servings. If you eat the M&M's, you are left with one more serving of carbohydrate to add to your diet for the day.

Please note that I do not advocate eating M&M's for weight loss. But let's get real. We all have days when we just need to give in to a craving. The M&M's example shows that even if you decide to indulge a bit, and eat a food that is relatively low in nutrients, you can still manage to stay within the program without feeling you have fallen off the wagon.

It's the mentality of "Oops, I ate something bad. I might as well continue to binge and go off my diet" that leads so many people to believe that diets don't work. I agree that eating "perfectly" healthily every day can be a challenge. That's why I designed the F-Factor Diet to accommodate indulgences every once in a while.

As long as you follow the basic principles of "fiber and protein at every meal," you will see that you can enjoy an occasional treat while continuing to lose weight and feel great.

## The Best Carbohydrates to Add to Your Diet for Continued Weight Loss

Although you can enjoy just about any food on Step 2, when considering which 3 carbohydrates to add to your day, there clearly are some choices that are better than others. While you can choose simple carbohydrates like white bread, chocolate, and chips, these foods will not provide you with long-term satiety. In fact, eating these foods may cause you to feel hungry soon after— leading you to eat more later on.

On the other hand, if you are looking for foods that are filling and keep you satisfied, then aim for carbohydrates loaded with fiber. Fiber helps to curb your appetite and keep you feeling fuller. Complex carbohydrates filled with fiber are digested gradually, provide an even blood sugar level, and serve as a constant fuel supply for the body and brain. Also, the more fiber a food contains, the less digestible carbohydrate it has, and the less effect it will have on filling up your glycogen stores.

Say you choose to add a piece of bread to your diet as 1 of the 3 carbo-hydrates. Do you choose white bread or whole wheat? A look at the labels reveals:

| NUTRITION FACTS | NUTRITION FACTS |
| --- | --- |
| White Bread: | Whole-Wheat Bread: |
| Serving Size: 1 slice | Serving Size: 1 slice |
| 80 Calories | 80 Calories |
| 15 g Carbohydrate | 15 g Carbohydrate |
| 0 g Fiber | 5 g Fiber |
| Net Carbohydrate 15 g | Net Carbohydrate 10 g |

The whole-wheat bread slice is clearly the better choice. Not only does it have more fiber, and therefore fewer net carbs, but also it will take longer to digest than the white bread, leading you to feel fuller longer. The longer you feel full after a meal, the less likely you are to overeat at the next meal.

Let's take a look at two fruit choices:

| NUTRITION FACTS | NUTRITION FACTS |
| --- | --- |
| **Blueberries:** | **Raisins:** |
| Serving Size: ¾ cup | Serving size: 2 tablespoons |
| 60 calories | 60 calories |
| 15 g Carbohydrate | 15 g Carbohydrate |
| 5 g Fiber | 1 g Fiber |
| Net Carbohydrate 10 g | Net Carbohydrate 14 g |

Although both blueberries and raisins have 15 grams of carbohydrate per serving, the fiber content varies drastically. The blueberries contain 5 grams of fiber while the raisins contain only 1 gram. The fewer grams of net carbohydrate results in a slower fill of your glycogen stores, which is one of the factors leading to fat storage. In addition, the fiber in the blueberries adds bulk, which is why you get a ¾ cup portion versus a mere 2 tbsp. of raisins for the same 15 grams of carbohydrates.

The point is that when you choose to add in the 3 carbohydrates to Step 2, aim for those with the most fiber. It is the fiber that will help keep you feeling full while losing weight.

Never before have there been so many high-fiber foods on the market. Aside from foods naturally high in fiber, like fruits, vegetables, whole grains, and beans, food manufacturers are introducing more high-fiber foods to the marketplace. In 2006 alone, about 670 new food items appeared making high-fiber claims on their packages. Some items are newly formulated while others simply have new packaging that makes a high-fiber claim. Available packaged foods high in fiber include:

F-Factor Fiber/Protein products
Planters nuts
Fig Newtons
Kellogg's Eggo Nutri-Grain whole-wheat waffles
Dannon Oikos Triple Zero Greek nonfat yogurt
Stove Top stuffing
Bob's Red Mill Wheat Rolled (flakes)
V8 Vegetable Juice
Barilla ProteinPlus pasta

Kellogg's Frosted Mini Wheats cereals
Thomas' High Fiber English muffins
Wonder whole-wheat bread

Never has it been easier to meet your fiber needs while eating healthy, delicious foods that are accessible and widely available.

## Step 2 Journal

Packaged foods have nutrition facts labels, so it is easy to see the carbohydrate and fiber content of these foods. For foods that lack nutrition facts labels, such as fresh fruits, vegetables, and meats, you should use the exchange lists in Chapter 3 to determine serving size or carbohydrate and fiber content. This information is necessary for filling out your Step 2 journals. Enclosed in this chapter is a Step 2 journal page. Make at least 30 copies, and fill out 1 journal page per day. Alternatively, in the F-Factor App, select Step 2 on your profile to access the Step 2 journal.

### How Long to Stay on Step 2

Because of the addition of carbohydrates in Step 2, you will feel more energized than you did in Step 1. As you learned in Chapter 4, carbohydrates are used for energy. You will stay on Step 2 until you reach your goal weight, when you will go on to Step 3 (maintenance).

You should lose approximately 1 to 2 pounds a week on Step 2. You've heard it before, and it's true: you didn't put the weight on overnight, and you are not going to lose it overnight.

You may wish you could lose up to 10 pounds a week, but keep in mind that slow, gradual weight loss is more likely to be permanent. Losing weight at a steady pace represents a healthy lifestyle change rather than a short-term diet fad. The F-Factor Diet not only helps you lose weight but also, more important, helps you keep it off.

| Date: | | Carb | Fiber |
|---|---|---|---|
| **BREAKFAST** | | | |
| | | | |
| | | | |
| | | | |
| | | | |
| **LUNCH** | | | |
| | | | |
| | | | |
| | | | |
| | | | |
| **SNACK** | | | |
| | | | |
| **DINNER/SUPPER** | | | |
| | | | |
| | | | |
| | | | |
| | | | |
| **SNACK/DESSERT** | | | |
| | | | |

$$A - B = C$$
$$g - g = g$$

ingested carb    fiber

<75 g net carb/day

| | g | g |
|---|---|---|
| | A | B >35 g |

THE F-FACTOR DIET

# Foods Permitted on Step 2

*All* the foods allowed on Step 1 *plus* an additional 3 servings of carbohydrate of your choice:

## STARCH LIST

| | Serving Size | Carbs (g) | Fiber (g) |
|---|---|---|---|
| **BREAD** | | | |
| bagel, 4 oz | ¼ (1 oz) | 15 | 1 |
| biscuit, 2½ inches across | 1 | 15 | 1 |
| bread, reduced calorie | 2 slices | 15 | 1 |
| bread, white | 1 slice | 15 | 1 |
| bread, pumpernickel, rye | 1 slice | 15 | 2 |
| bread, whole-wheat | 1 slice | 15 | 2–6 |
| corn bread, 2-inch cube | 1 (2 oz) | 15 | 1 |
| English muffin | ½ | 15 | 1 |
| English muffin, whole-wheat | ½ | 15 | 2 |
| hot dog bun or hamburger bun | ½ | 15 | 1 |
| naan, 8 x 2 inch | ¼ | 15 | 1 |
| pancake, 4 inches across | 1 | 15 | 0 |
| pancake, whole-wheat | 1 | 15 | 2 |
| pita, 6 inches across | ½ | 15 | 1 |
| pita, whole-wheat, 6 inches across | ½ | 15 | 2 |
| roll, plain, small | 1 (1 oz) | 15 | 1 |
| raisin bread, unfrosted | 1 slice | 15 | 1 |
| stuffing, bread (prepared) | ⅓ cup | 15 | 1–2 |
| taco shell, 5 inches across | 2 | 15 | 1 |
| tortilla, corn or flour, 6 inches across | 1 | 15 | 1 |
| tortilla, flour, 10 inches across | ⅓ | 15 | 1 |
| waffle, 4-inch square | 1 | 15 | 1 |
| **CEREALS AND GRAINS** | | | |
| bran cereals | ½ cup | 15 | 5–14 |

| | Serving Size | Carbs (g) | Fiber (g) |
|---|---|---|---|
| bulgur | ½ cup | 15 | 4 |
| cereals, cooked | ½ cup | 15 | 2 |
| cereals, unsweetened, ready-to-eat | ¾ cup | 15 | 0–5 |
| cornmeal (dry) | 2½ tbsp. | 15 | 1–2 |
| couscous | ⅓ cup | 15 | 1 |
| flour (dry) | 3 tbsp. | 15 | 1 |
| granola, low-fat | ¼ cup | 15 | 1–3 |
| Grape-Nuts | 3 tbsp. | 15 | 3 |
| grits (cooked) | ½ cup | 15 | 1 |
| kasha (cooked) | ½ cup | 15 | 2 |
| millet (cooked) | ⅓ cup | 15 | 2 |
| muesli | ¼ cup | 15 | 2 |
| oats (dry) | ½ cup | 15 | 3 |
| pasta (cooked) | ½ cup | 15 | 1 |
| puffed cereal | 1½ cups | 15 | 1 |
| quinoa (cooked) | ⅓ cup | 15 | 2 |
| rice, white (cooked) | ⅓ cup | 15 | 1 |
| rice, brown (cooked) | ⅓ cup | 15 | 2 |
| shredded wheat | ⅓ cup | 15 | 2 |
| sugar-frosted cereal | ½ cup | 15 | 0–3 |
| wheat germ | ¼ cup | 15 | 4 |

## STARCHY VEGETABLES

| | Serving Size | Carbs (g) | Fiber (g) |
|---|---|---|---|
| baked beans | ⅓ cup | 15 | 4 |
| corn | ½ cup | 15 | 3 |
| corn on cob, 6 in. | 1 long | 15 | 2 |
| French-fried potatoes (oven-baked) | 1 cup | 15 | 2 |
| mixed vegetables with corn, peas | 1 cup | 15 | 3 |
| peas, green | ½ cup | 15 | 4 |
| plaintain | ⅓ cup | 15 | 0 |
| potato, boiled | ½ cup | 15 | 2 |
| potato, baked with skin | ¼ large (3 oz) | 15 | 3 |
| potato, mashed | ½ cup | 15 | 2 |
| squash, winter (acorn, butternut, pumpkin) | 1 cup | 15 | 4 |
| yam, sweet potato, plain with skin | ½ cup | 15 | 4 |

| | Serving Size | Carbs (g) | Fiber (g) |
|---|---|---|---|
| **CRACKERS AND SNACKS** | | | |
| animal crackers | 8 | 15 | 0 |
| chow mein noodles | ½ cup | 15 | 1 |
| crackers, round butter type | 6 | 15 | 0 |
| graham crackers, 2½ in. square | 3 | 15 | 1 |
| matzoh | ¾ oz | 15 | 1 |
| oyster crackers | 20 | 15 | 0 |
| popcorn (popped, no fat added) | 3 cups | 15 | 3 |
| pretzels | ¾ oz | 15 | 0 |
| rice cakes, 4 inches across | 2 | 15 | 0 |
| saltine-type crackers | 6 | 15 | 0 |
| sandwich crackers, cheese or peanut butter filling | 3 | 15 | 0 |
| snack chips, fat-free or baked (tortilla, potato) | 8 (¾ oz) | 15 | 2 |
| whole-wheat crackers, no fat added | 2–4 (¾ oz) | 15 | 2 |
| **BEANS, PEAS AND LENTILS** | | | |
| beans/peas (garbanzo, pinto, kidney, white, split) | ½ cup | 15 | 6 |
| hummus | ⅓ cup | 15 | 2 |
| lima beans | ½ cup | 15 | 5 |
| lentils (cooked) | ½ cup | 15 | 8 |
| miso | 3 tbsp. | 15 | 3 |

# FRUIT LIST

| **FRUIT** | | | |
|---|---|---|---|
| apple, unpeeled, small | 1 (4 oz) | 15 | 3 |
| applesauce, unsweetened | ½ cup | 15 | 1 |
| apples, dried | 4 rings | 15 | 2 |
| apricots, fresh | 4 whole | 15 | 3 |
| apricots, dried | 8 halves | 15 | 2 |
| apricots, canned | ½ cup | 15 | 2 |

| | Serving Size | Carbs (g) | Fiber (g) |
|---|---|---|---|
| banana, small | 1 (4 oz) | 15 | 2 |
| blackberries | 1 cup | 15 | 8 |
| blueberries | ¾ cup | 15 | 5 |
| cantaloupe, small | 1 cup cubes | 15 | 1 |
| cherries, fresh | 12 | 15 | 2 |
| cherries, sweet, canned | ½ cup | 15 | 1 |
| dates | 3 small/1 large | 15 | 2 |
| figs, dried | 2 | 15 | 2 |
| fruit cocktail | ½ cup | 15 | 1 |
| grapefruit, large | ½ | 15 | 2 |
| grapes | 15 | 15 | 1 |
| honeydew melon | 1 slice | 15 | 1 |
| kiwi | 1 | 15 | 3 |
| mandarin oranges, canned | ¾ cup | 15 | 1 |
| mango, small | ½ fruit or ½ cup | 15 | 1 |
| nectarine, medium | 1 | 15 | 2 |
| orange, medium | 1 (6½ oz) | 15 | 3 |
| papaya | ½ fruit | 15 | 3 |
| peach, fresh | 1 | 15 | 2 |
| peaches, canned | ½ cup | 15 | 2 |
| pear, large, fresh | ½ (4 oz) | 15 | 4 |
| pears, canned | ½ cup | 15 | 2 |
| pineapple, fresh | ¾ cup | 15 | 2 |
| pineapple, canned | ½ cup | 15 | 1 |
| plums, small | 2 | 15 | 2 |
| raisins | 2 tbsp. | 15 | 1 |
| raspberries | 1 cup | 15 | 8 |
| strawberries | 1¼ cup | 15 | 4 |
| tangerines, small | 2 | 15 | 2 |
| watermelon | 1¼ cup | 15 | 1 |

**FRUIT JUICE**

| | Serving Size | Carbs (g) | Fiber (g) |
|---|---|---|---|
| apple juice/cider | ½ cup | 15 | 0 |
| cranberry juice cocktail | ⅓ cup | 15 | 0 |

| | Serving Size | Carbs (g) | Fiber (g) |
|---|---|---|---|
| cranberry juice cocktail, reduced-calorie | 1 cup | 15 | 0 |
| fruit juice blends, 100% juice | ⅓ cup | 15 | 0 |
| grape juice | ⅓ cup | 15 | 0 |
| grapefruit juice | ½ cup | 15 | 0 |
| orange juice | ½ cup | 15 | 0 |
| pineapple juice | ½ cup | 15 | 0 |
| prune juice | ⅓ cup | 15 | 1 |

## MILK LIST

### FAT-FREE AND LOW-FAT MILK

12 grams of carbohydrate (count as 15 grams of carbohydrate), 8 grams of protein, 0–3 grams of fat, and 90 calories

| | | | |
|---|---|---|---|
| fat-free milk | 1 cup | 15 | 0 |
| 1% milk | 1 cup | 15 | 0 |
| 2% milk | 1 cup | 15 | 0 |
| buttermilk, low-fat or fat-free | 1 cup | 15 | 0 |
| evaporated fat-free milk | ½ cup | 15 | 0 |
| fat-free dry milk | ⅓ cup dry | 15 | 0 |
| soy milk, low-fat or fat-free | 1 cup | 15 | 1 |
| yogurt, fat-free, sweetened with no-calorie sweetener | ⅔ cup (6 oz) | 15 | 0 |
| yogurt, plain, fat-free | ¾ cup | 15 | 0 |
| yogurt, plain reduced-fat | ⅔ cup/ 6 oz | 15 | 0 |
| soy milk | 1 cup | 15 | 2 |

## Step 2 Guidelines

### BREAKFAST

Choose 1 from the options below. Option to pair with additional side.

### HIGH FIBER CEREAL AND LEAN PROTEIN:

½ cup All-Bran Original, Fiber One Original or Nature's Path SmartBran, or ⅓ cup All-Bran Bran Buds cereal and 1 serving of fruit (2 total servings of carbohydrate) with either:

- 1 cup 1–2% cottage cheese
- 6 ounces 0% fat Greek or Icelandic yogurt
- 1 cup unsweetened almond milk, skim or 2% milk

## HIGH-FIBER CRACKERS OR TOAST AND LEAN PROTEIN:

Four high-fiber crackers, such as GG Bran Crispbreads or 1 piece whole-wheat toast (1 serving carbohydrate) with any protein from the very lean or lean meat and meat substitutes list in Chapter 3. Examples include, but are not limited to:

- 2–4 egg whites, Egg Beaters, or egg and egg white combination (1 egg yolk with 2 egg whites)
  - ➤ *Omelets/eggs can be made with your favorite vegetables and nonfat or low-fat cheese*
- ½ cup–1 cup 1–2% cottage cheese
- 2–4 ounces smoked salmon with 2 Tbsp low fat cream cheese

## FIBER AND PROTEIN ON-THE-GO:
- High fiber/high protein smoothie or shake (see recipe on pp. 182 and 219 for example)
- F-Factor Fiber/Protein Bar

## OPTIONAL SIDES:
- 2 ounces turkey bacon, Canadian bacon, low-fat sausage, smoked salmon, or any lean or very lean protein
- serving of fruit
- nonstarchy vegetables

## LUNCH

Choose 1 from each category. Option to pair with 2–4 high-fiber crackers, or a whole-wheat bread or wrap to make a sandwich (look at nutrition label for carb and fiber content—will be 1–2 servings carbohydrate)

## FIBER:
- Garden salad with oil and vinegar (no more than 2 tsp oil), light dressing, or squeeze of fresh lemon
- 1–2 cups fresh vegetables (crudités, salad, etc.)

- 1 cup gazpacho, vegetable soup, miso soup, or consommé with vegetables and chicken (no rice, pasta, potatoes, beans, or cream)

## Protein:

3–6 ounces of any protein from the very lean or lean meat and meat substitutes list in Chapter 3. Examples include, but are not limited to:

- Tuna salad, chicken salad, or crab salad (prepared with nonfat mayonnaise)
- Tuna, salmon, crab meat, shrimp, or lobster
- Lunch meat: sliced turkey, lean ham, roast beef
- Poultry (no skin), lean beef
- Cottage cheese, part-skim mozzarella cheese
- Lite tofu

## SNACK

Pair protein with at least one fruit, vegetable, or whole-grain item when snacking. Avoid sugars—cookies, candy, colas, and other sugary treats give you instant energy but are followed by an energy crash. Suggestions include:

- 1 ounce of nuts and 1 piece of fruit
- 4 high-fiber crackers with 2 tbsp. peanut butter
- 4 high-fiber crackers with 2 ounces of low-fat cheese of lean meat (i.e., 2 Laughing Cow Light cheese wedges or 2 ounces of sliced turkey or ham) and an apple
- 1 container 0% fat Greek or Icelandic yogurt with ⅓ cup All-Bran Bran Buds
- 2 cups of air-fat popcorn sprinkled with Parmesan cheese
- 1 piece of string cheese with one piece of fruit
- 1 apple with 2 tbsp. peanut butter
- ½ turkey, grilled chicken, or ham sandwich on whole-wheat bread with lettuce, tomato, and mustard
- ½ cup chickpeas, chopped tomatoes, onions, and cucumbers with balsamic vinegar
- 2 tbsp. hummus, 10 baby carrots
- ½ whole-wheat pita or English muffin with 1 ounce melted cheese and sliced turkey

- Whole-wheat pita pizza (on ½ whole-wheat pita spread 2 tbsp. pizza sauce, and ¼ cup shredded low-fat mozzarella, and toast until cheese melts)
- 2–4 high-fiber crackers with fat-free cream cheese and smoked salmon
- ½ cup chicken, tuna or egg white salad made with chopped celery and onion and nonfat mayonnaise on a whole-wheat English muffin or with high-fiber crackers
- ½ cup cottage cheese with fiber cereal or high-fiber crackers and 1 mini-box of raisins
- Fiber/Protein bar or Fiber/Protein shake

## DINNER

Choose 1 from each course/category:

### APPETIZERS/SIDES:
- Salad with low-fat or nonfat dressing
- Soup (broth-based, made without cream, potatoes, pasta, rice, or beans)

### VEGETABLES:
Any vegetables (from the nonstarchy vegetables list) steamed, sautéed, or grilled (prepared with minimum oil)

### MAIN COURSE:
4–6 ounces of any protein from the very lean or lean lists in Chapter 3. Examples include, but are not limited to:

- Beef: lean cuts such as sirloin, tenderloin, flank steak, ground round, and top round
- Poultry: chicken or turkey (no skin), Cornish hen (no skin), duck (well drained of fat, no skin), ground chicken, or turkey breast (99% lean)
- Seafood: all types of fish and shellfish (broiled, grilled, steamed, poached—not fried)
- Pork: boiled ham, Canadian bacon, tenderloin, center loin chop
- Veal: chop, leg cutlet, top round
- Lunch meat: sliced turkey, ham, roast beef
- Cheese (fat-free or low-fat): American, cheddar, 1% fat cottage cheese, fat-free or low-fat cream cheese, feta, mozzarella, Parmesan, provolone, and ricotta

## DESSERT (OPTIONAL):

- Sugar-free Jell-O
- 1 Tofutti Chocolate Fudge Treat
- ½ cup Arctic Zero Creamy Pints
- sugar-free ice pop
- diet hot chocolate
- 1 small serving of fruit
- 1 serving New Pop Skinless Popcorn, Skinny Pop, or other low-calorie popcorn

## CRACKERS OR TOAST:

Four high-fiber crackers, such as GG Bran Crispbreads, or 1 piece whole-wheat toast with either:

- 2–4 egg whites (scrambled, omelet, hard-boiled)
- Egg Beaters
- Eggs and egg white combination (1 egg yolk with 2 egg whites)
- 1 cup 1–2% cottage cheese

*Omelets/eggs can be made with your favorite vegetables and nonfat or low-fat cheese*

# A Sample Menu Plan and Corresponding Journal for Step 2

## BREAKFAST

The F-Factor Diet Breakfast Sandwich:
Thomas' English muffin light multigrain topped with
    Canadian bacon (1 slice), 1 fried egg, 1 slice low-fat cheese
1 orange

## LUNCH

turkey burger on whole-wheat bun with lettuce, onion, tomato
1 cup baby carrots
diet iced tea or coffee

## MIDAFTERNOON SNACK

4 GG Bran Crispbreads
2 tbsp. PB2 powdered peanut butter

# EXAMPLE OF A STEP 2 JOURNAL ENTRY

| Date: Monday, June 1 | Carb | Fiber |
|---|---|---|
| **BREAKFAST** The F-Factor Diet Breakfast Sandwich | | |
| Thomas' English muffin light multigrain | 25 | 8 |
| 1 slice Canadian bacon | 0 | 0 |
| 1 egg | 0 | 0 |
| 1 slice low-fat cheese | 0 | 0 |
| 1 orange | 15 | 3 |
| **LUNCH** | | |
| turkey burger | 0 | 0 |
| whole-wheat bun | 15 | 2 |
| 2 slices tomato, Romaine lettuce, sliced onion | 0 | 2 |
| 1 cup baby carrots | 0 | 4 |
| diet iced tea | 0 | 0 |
| **SNACK** | | |
| 4 GG Bran Crispbreads | 24 | 16 |
| 2 tbsp. PB2 powdered peanut butter | 5 | 2 |
| **DINNER/SUPPER** | | |
| 6 oz. New York strip steak | 0 | 0 |
| 1 cup grilled asparagus | 0 | 6 |
| 1/2 baked sweet potato | 15 | 4 |
| 1 cup salad greens with 1 tbsp. vinaigrette | 0 | 2 |
| 1 glass red wine | 2 | 0 |
| **SNACK/DESSERT** | | |
| Sugar-free Jell-O with 1 tbsp. fat-free Cool Whip | 0 | 0 |
| **A − B = C** <br> 101 g − 49 g = 52 g <br> ingested carb / fiber / (52) <br> <75 g net carb/day | 101 g <br><br> A | 49 g <br><br> B >35 g |

### DINNER

1 6 oz New York strip steak

½ baked sweet potato

1 cup grilled or steamed asparagus

1 cup salad greens with 1 tbsp. vinaigrette dressing

1 glass red wine

### DESSERT

Sugar-free Jell-O with fat-free Cool Whip, or So Delicious Dairy Free CocoWhip!

## Tips for Breakfast

1. Avoid sugar.
2. Limit caffeine. One cup of coffee can kick-start your day, but more than three cups and you are likely to spiral into caffeine withdrawal and need more coffee to pep you up. You may also sleep poorly at night and wake up tired the next morning.
3. Choose foods with a mix of protein and fiber to maintain blood sugar and energy levels throughout the morning. Examples include:
   - egg-white omelet with low-fat cheese and chopped vegetables plus 2–4 high-fiber crackers, or 1 piece of whole-wheat toast
   - fiber cereal with ½ cup cottage cheese, or 1 cup yogurt, skim milk, unsweetened almond milk, or soymilk with ¾ cup blueberries
   - 1 slice whole-wheat toast with 1 tbsp. of peanut butter and ½ grapefruit

## Tips for Lunch

What and how much you eat at lunch can make or break your energy level by midafternoon. Some good rules of thumb are:

1. Keep it light. A light meal of 500 calories or less will fuel your energy without leaving you drowsy.
2. Keep it low-fat. Fatty meals will prime you for a nap rather than a get-things-done afternoon.

3. Choose foods with a mix of protein and fiber to maintain blood sugar and energy levels.

Lunch examples include:

- sandwiches made with whole-wheat bread and low-fat cold cuts (turkey, roast beef, lean ham) with lettuce, tomato, and mustard and a piece of fruit
- a large salad with as many vegetables as you would like topped with grilled chicken, shrimp, or turkey, ½ cup of beans (high in fiber!), and low-fat or nonfat dressing and 2 high-fiber crackers
- a bowl of bean soup and a side salad, plus fiber crackers with low-fat cheese
- miso soup, a side salad with ginger dressing and sashimi
- hot and sour soup, and steamed Chinese mixed vegetables with shrimp, chicken, or lobster

## Tips for Snacking

Very few of us can resist snacking, and you don't need to if you snack intelligently. In fact, maintaining high energy levels throughout the day requires frequent stops for fuel and nutrients. Always eat an afternoon snack to keep your energy levels up so you can get through the rest of your day. In addition, having a snack keeps you from being overly ravenous at dinner. Remember, when it comes to snacks:

1. *Simplify:* A nutritious snack must be convenient. That is, it must be readily available, take little time to prepare, and taste great.
2. Eat at least one fruit, vegetable, or whole-grain item when snacking, plus one or more of the following:
   - nuts
   - nonfat milk products, such as yogurt, low-fat cottage cheese, or low-fat cheese
   - cooked beans or extra-lean meats, which are a great source of iron, the energy-boosting mineral that many women don't get enough of
3. *Plan ahead.* Pack your purse, briefcase, desk drawer, and office refrigerator with fresh fruit, baby carrots, fiber crackers, dried fruit, string cheese,

fiber cereal, and yogurt. Eat a nutritious snack at the first sign of hunger to avoid overeating the wrong foods once you're ravenous.

4. Skipping an afternoon snack will cause you to overeat at dinner, which is the *worst* time of day to overeat! At night, you are less active and therefore less likely to burn calories. So eat most of your calories before dinner, when you are more likely to burn them off through activity.

## Tips for Dinner

Focus on eating lean protein and vegetables. At dinner, eat carbohydrates such as rice, potatoes, bread, and pasta in moderation; these are easy to over-eat—a single serving is much less than you are used to! Extra carbohydrates at dinner are more likely to be converted into fat than those eaten earlier in the day. Keep that in mind when preparing or ordering dinner. Some good examples of dinner include:

1. Tossed green salad with nonfat dressing, 5 oz fillet of sole (or any lean fish), ½ baked sweet potato and steamed asparagus, 1 piece of fruit

2. Mixed green salad or a cup of soup (no cream or added starch), 5 oz grilled filet mignon, 1 cup sautéed spinach, sautéed mushrooms and on-ions, 1 cup strawberries

3. 5 oz grilled skinless chicken breast, ½ cup whole-wheat pasta with ½ cup vegetables and low-sugar tomato sauce, 2 tbsp. Parmesan cheese, 1 cup sliced pears

Continue to keep a journal every day. This will increase your awareness of the foods you eat and help to ensure that you are keeping your carbo-hydrate intake within Step 2 parameters (below 75 grams net carbohydrate per day).

Finally, make sure you drink enough water throughout the day. The Insti-tute of Medicine determined that an adequate intake (AI) for men is roughly about 13 cups (3 liters) of total beverages a day. The AI for women is about 9 cups (2.2 liters) of total beverages a day. Water is the number one component of the human body. Water makes up 50 to 60 percent of your weight, and plays a vital role in regulating body temperature, transporting nutrients and oxygen, and cushioning joints and organs. Not drinking enough fluids, on the other hand, has been linked to gallstones, bladder cancer, blood clots, irregular heartbeat, and impaired mental focus.

Getting enough fluid is not only crucial to your health but, if you are trying to lose weight, keeping hydrated may be the key to your success. Symptoms of dehydration include fatigue, headaches, and muscle cramping. These symptoms are similar to those of hunger and may easily be confused with each other. Often people eat in response to these symptoms, thinking that they need food in order to feel better, when in fact all they need is some fluids. The next time you feel tired or cranky, before you reach for a snack, first drink a bottle of zero-calorie water to see if the symptoms go away.

You should aim for at least 8 8-oz. glasses of water a day. Drink more if you exercise intensely or if you consume coffee or tea, which both act as diuretics and aggravate dehydration.

**You have already achieved a great deal and are on your way to even better results in terms of how you look and feel. Keep up the good work!**

## Frequently Asked Questions on Step 2

**QUESTION:** What is considered a high-fiber carbohydrate?
**ANSWER:** A high-fiber carbohydrate contains 5 grams of fiber or more per serving. Foods that contain 2.5–4.9 grams of fiber per serving are considered a good source of fiber, while less than 2.5 grams is considered a low-fiber food.

**High-fiber:** 5 grams or more per serving
**Good source of fiber:** 2–4.9 grams per serving
**Low-fiber:** less than 2 grams per serving

But keep in mind that high fiber content alone does not make a food healthy. The ratio of fiber to carbohydrate also matters. For example, there is a big difference between a food that contains 30 grams of carbohydrate and 10 grams of fiber and one that contains 30 grams of carbohydrate and only

1 gram of fiber. When a food contains a lot of carbohydrate and virtually no fiber, it is primarily refined (white flours and sugars). On the other hand, if a food has a lot of carbohydrate but also a high fiber content, then the carbohydrates in the food are typically complex. Scan food labels for bread and cereal products listing whole grain or whole wheat as the first ingredient.

The more fiber a food has, the more slowly the food is digested, resulting in a slower rise and fall of blood sugar. High-fiber foods also cause you to feel fuller longer on fewer calories. *Aim for foods that not only have more than 5 grams of fiber but also have a close ratio of carbohydrates to fiber.* For example, the high-fiber crackers I recommend have 6 grams of carbohydrate and 4 grams of fiber, resulting in 2 grams net carbs. Most foods contain more carbohydrate than fiber so a good rule of thumb is to *look for those with no more than 45 grams of carbohydrate and at least 5 grams of fiber per serving.*

QUESTION: Do I have to add all 3 servings of carbohydrates on Step 2? What if I feel satisfied with just adding 1 or 2 servings a day?

ANSWER: By far, this is the question I hear most often from patients. After losing weight on Step 1, many people hesitate to add in more food on Step 2, fearing they will not continue to lose weight as effectively. It is true that by adding more foods to your diet, you will not lose as much weight per week as you did during Step 1. But in the long run, *adding* additional high-fiber carbohydrates will enable you to continue to drop unwanted pounds while feeling full and satisfied.

Step 1 is very low in calories (average caloric intake is anywhere from 900 to 1100 calories per day). When you drastically reduce caloric intake for an extended period of time, your body thinks it is starving and goes into self-preservation mode. Your metabolism will slow down, so that you won't quickly burn the calories you are consuming. If you are trying to lose weight, slowing down your metabolism is the last thing you want to do. Therefore, by adding in more food in Step 2, you are guaranteeing that your body won't go into starvation mode and will continue to burn calories effectively.

Because Step 2 adds just 3 servings of carbohydrate (approximately 240 calories), you can be assured that you are not eating an excessive amount of calories that would impede further weight loss. In fact, adding the 3 servings of high-fiber carbohydrates will enable you to lose weight more effectively than if you did not add them.

**QUESTION:** I don't want to be left out when my co-workers order in lunch. What can I do to join them without consuming more calories than I want to eat?

**ANSWER:** When you call in your order, ask about healthier alternatives that may not be listed on the menu. Most restaurants can grill a chicken breast and serve it over a chopped green salad. Ask for oil and vinegar on the side and a small whole-wheat roll. See Chapter 9 for more suggestions of good choices at a variety of ethnic and fast-food restaurants.

**QUESTION:** I heard you can drink alcohol on this diet. Why is it that I can drink alcohol on the F-Factor Diet and still lose weight?

**ANSWER:** You heard it right! F-Factor was created to help you lose weight without disrupting your lifestyle.

For years, researchers have debated whether alcohol is good or bad for you. It is safe to say that alcohol is both a tonic and a poison. Moderate drinking seems to be good for the heart and circulatory system, and probably protects against type 2 diabetes and gallstones. Heavy drinking, on the other hand, is linked to liver disease, heart disease, and an increased risk of breast cancer and other cancers.

As far as the relationship between moderate drinking and weight gain goes, the jury is still out. Many diet and weight-loss programs caution about alcohol consumption, stating that wine, beer, and spirits lead to weight gain by increasing the appetite while lowering inhibitions, a deadly combination that leads to overeating and poor food choices. However, research increasingly suggests that moderate consumption does not represent a dietary risk factor for developing obesity. In a 2004 study conducted at the Departments of Nutrition and Epidemiology, Harvard School of Public Health, researchers reported that one drink a day did not contribute to weight gain, particularly in women. In fact, alcohol may actually increase your metabolism slightly so that you burn more calories.

To help you decide what to order at the bar, here are some of the most and least caloric alcoholic beverages with their calorie, carbohydrate and fiber counts.

Mixed drinks generally contain the most calories because of the juice and sugar:

| MOST CALORIC DRINKS | CALORIES | CARBS | FIBER |
|---|---|---|---|
| frozen daiquiri | 400 | 45 g | 0 g |
| margarita | 330 | 20 g | 0 g |
| amaretto sour | 300 | 30 g | 0 g |
| eggnog | 300 | 30 g | 0 g |
| piña colada | 250 | 30 g | 0 g |
| vodka cranberry | 250 | 30 g | 0 g |
| gin/vodka tonic | 200 | 20 g | 0 g |
| beer, regular | 150–200 | 10–15 g | 0 g |

| LEAST CALORIC DRINKS | CALORIES | CARBS | FIBER |
|---|---|---|---|
| Bloody Mary | 120 | 5 g | 1 g |
| red or white wine, 5 oz | 80–100 | 2 g | 0 g |
| distilled liquors (whiskey, gin, rum, vodka), 90 proof, 1 oz | 100 | 0 g | 0 g |
| gin/vodka and diet tonic | 100 | 0 g | 0 g |
| rum and Diet Coke | 100 | 0 g | 0 g |
| Champagne | 100 | 0 g | 0 g |
| low-carb beer | 99 | 3 g | 0 g |
| white wine spritzer | 75 | 1 g | 0 g |

Many people enjoy a glass of wine with dinner or a drink when they're out with friends at a social gathering. This was an important fact I kept in mind when creating the F-Factor Diet. The reason most diets are temporary is that they are too restrictive, forcing you to excise your favorite foods and often making you cut out alcohol as well. So I knew that if people were truly to embrace the F-Factor as a lifestyle, then moderate alcohol consumption had to be a part of the program.

The key is to make choices. For example, when you have a glass of wine with dinner, you may choose to skip dessert. Although wine and spirits contain minimal carbohydrates, count each glass as one of your carbohydrate servings in Steps 2 and 3. This will help you keep your overall calories in check.

The bottom line is that a calorie is a calorie, and a 100-calorie alcoholic beverage constitutes only a small portion of the total amount of calories you consume. However, what you need to keep in mind is that these are "empty calories" as alcohol has no nutritional value. Thus, it is important to limit yourself to one serving per day for women and two for men—the current health guidelines from the U.S. Department of Agriculture—so that you avoid filling up on alcohol at the expense of nutritious foods and beverages.

## CHAPTER 8

## STEP 3: MAINTENANCE—EATING FOR LIFE

*My doctor told me to stop having intimate dinners for four.*
*Unless there are three other people.*

—ORSON WELLES

CONGRATULATIONS on making it to the maintenance phase. You have learned and applied the principles of the F-Factor Diet and are looking and feeling better than you have in years. You are now ready to begin Step 3, a phase you'll stay with forever—for the rest of your healthy life.

## Add 3 More Servings of Carbohydrate

At this point, you will add another 3 servings of carbohydrate (that is, an additional 45 grams) to your eating plan on Step 2. Your net carbohydrate intake on Step 3 will be 125 grams or less per day (on average), with a continued fiber intake of at least 35 grams.

By now you've learned a new way of eating that enables you to eat plenty of fresh fruits and vegetables, lots of lean protein and dairy, and even moderate amounts of fat. You eat carbohydrates, but find that you gravitate toward those that contain fiber because of its many health benefits and the role it plays in helping you feel satisfied. Eating foods high in fiber is what has enabled you to lose weight without feeling hungry. You now have an entirely new outlook on food. Even a small portion of pasta (eaten Italian style as a first course or a side dish) isn't going to get you into trouble. In other words, you are able to eat just about anything, so long as you maintain your fiber intake. You know you'll be full and satisfied, so you won't even be tempted to go back to the refined carbohydrates and sugary foods that may have gotten you into trouble in the first place.

## A Sample Menu Plan and Corresponding Journal for Step 3

**BREAKFAST**

¾ cup All-Bran Complete Wheat Flakes Cereal with 1 cup skim milk

1 small banana

coffee or tea

**LUNCH**

1 cup black bean soup topped with

1 oz shredded reduced-fat cheddar cheese

salad with 3 oz grilled chicken and 1 tbsp. vinaigrette

2 high-fiber crackers, such as GG Bran Crispbreads

**MIDAFTERNOON SNACK**

1 F-Factor Fiber/Protein Bar

1 small skim cappuccino

**DINNER**

takeout rotisserie chicken dinner:

1 cup salad greens with 1 tbsp. vinaigrette

¼ BBQ chicken, breast meat, no skin

1 cup steamed vegetables

1 12 oz beer

**DESSERT**

1 cup skim milk

2 small (1¼-inch diameter) chocolate chip cookies

## Tips to Stay Motivated

We all have our tough moments—occasions when it would be easy to forget about fiber and fall prey to fattening food.

Bad eating habits, such as the midday munchies, are hard to break. Holiday parties filled with festive, fattening food are also a challenge. My clients often ask me what to do when these situations arise. Because everyone faces these dieting dilemmas, this chapter will address questions many of you may have and offer answers for successfully getting through those diet pitfalls.

### Dealing with Midday Munchies

You know the feeling: you're working at your desk and as four o'clock rolls around, you get an overwhelming craving for a snack. So you head for the vending machine and get yourself something to eat.

An afternoon snack isn't necessarily a bad thing. In fact, it is natural and healthy. A few hours after eating lunch, your blood sugars begin to come down, causing you to feel hungry and need a pick-me-up to get through the rest of the day. Eating a sensible snack will supply you with needed fuel and also help to prevent overeating at dinner. A high-fiber, high-protein snack will not only provide you with energy but since it is slowly digested it will also help avoid your arriving at dinner overly ravenous. If you eat lunch at 12:00 and you don't sit down for dinner until 7:00, you have gone seven hours without eating. No wonder you can't help but eat half the breadbasket while reading the menu. On the other hand, if you had eaten a snack, you might still be hungry by the time dinner rolled around, but not so ravenous that control would go out the window.

An afternoon snack can also aid weight loss by providing you with energy for your after-work exercise session. If you attempt to work out on an empty stomach, you may feel too fatigued and skip the workout altogether.

So what should you snack on? Avoid foods that give you an instant rush but leave you hungry soon after, like refined carbohydrates and sugary foods.

THE F-FACTOR DIET

| Date: Monday, June 11 | Carb | Fiber |
|---|---|---|
| **BREAKFAST** | | |
| ¾ cup All-Bran Complete Wheat Flakes Cereal | 24 | 5 |
| 1 small banana | 15 | 2 |
| 1 cup skim milk | 15 | 0 |
| **LUNCH** | | |
| 1 cup black bean soup topped with | 15 | 6 |
| 1 oz. shredded reduced-fat cheddar cheese | 0 | 0 |
| salad with 3 oz grilled chicken and | 0 | 2 |
| 1 tbsp. vinaigrette | 0 | 0 |
| 2 GG Bran Crispbreads | 12 | 8 |
| **SNACK** | | |
| 1 F-Factor Fiber/Protein Bar | 25 | 20 |
| 1 small skim cappuccino | 15 | 0 |
| **DINNER/SUPPER** | | |
| ¼ BBQ chicken, breast meat, no skin | 0 | 0 |
| 1 cup steamed vegetables | 0 | 4 |
| 1 12 oz. beer | 13 | 0 |
| 1 cup salad greens with 1 tbsp. vinaigrette | 0 | 2 |
| | | |
| **SNACK/DESSERT** | | |
| 1 cup skim milk | 15 | 0 |
| 2 small (1½-inch diameter) chocolate chip cookies | 15 | 0 |
| | 134 g | 49 g |
| | A | B >35 g |

$$A - B = C$$
$$134\,g - 49\,g = 85\,g$$

(85 g)

ingested carb · fiber

<125 g net carb/day

Avoid candy bars, cookies, and chips. Instead, choose foods high in fiber and that have some protein too.

Remember, "Fiber and protein at every meal makes losing weight no big deal!"

A few healthy snack suggestions:

- **1 cup of edamame (soybeans).** A good source of soy protein and fiber, and like unshelled peanuts, these force you to take your time eating them. Edamame also come dry roasted like salted peanuts. But unlike peanuts, edamame are a good source of soy protein and are low in fat.
- **high-fiber cereal with skim milk.** Buy individual boxes of whole-grain cereal with bits of fruit, like raisin bran, and keep them stashed in your desk drawer.
- **whole-wheat crackers with peanut butter.** Peanut butter is a good source of protein, but is high in fat and calories; so be sure to limit yourself to no more than 2 tbsp. for a snack.
- **an apple with a piece of string cheese.** Apples are a crunchy and filling way to satisfy a sweet tooth. The string cheese is a low-fat source of protein that gives you the added benefit of some calcium.
- **1 ounce of nuts mixed with 2 tbsp. of raisins.** This is a great snack for people on the go. Put it into a baggie and carry it in your briefcase or purse. The mix of nuts with raisins not only provides you with protein and fiber but also will satisfy your craving for salty and sweet.
- **½ whole-wheat sandwich filled with turkey, lettuce, tomato, and mustard.** For a more filling snack, choose half a sandwich on whole-grain bread. Other lean protein substitutes for turkey include low-fat tuna salad, a slice of low-fat cheese, or grilled chicken.

## Staying on Track During the Holidays

For many of us, holidays are a nonstop feeding frenzy. With the seemingly inexhaustible supply of calorie-laden goodies at work, at parties, and at those never-ending family gatherings, it's no wonder the average American gains 5 to 7 pounds between Thanksgiving and New Year's. But holidays don't have to ruin your good intentions, especially if you plan ahead.

Before attending any holiday party, write down your food intentions before you go to the gathering. Giving yourself a clear plan will help you to stay focused. I also recommend that my clients have a high-fiber and protein snack right beforehand to fill them so they don't arrive ravenous. If you feel reasonably full before you arrive, the food served isn't such a big deal. You can simply have a taste and not blow your eating plans.

If there are appetizers, nibble on low-fat crudités like baby carrots and celery dipped in salsa, or healthful finger foods like grapes. Other healthy appetizers include ½ ounce of smoked salmon on a multigrain cracker, 1 to 2 whole-wheat pita triangles dipped in hummus, or a small handful of roasted almonds.

Avoid fattening chips, fried appetizers, and full-fat cheeses served on refined crackers. Another tip is to always hold a beverage in your hand. Holding a beverage will keep your hands occupied so they are less available to dip into some of the more fattening foods. Good beverage choices include a wine spritzer (70 calories), a glass of red or white wine (90 calories), and calorie-free beverages like water, iced tea, and seltzer.

When it comes to the main meal, fill up your plate with lean proteins (chicken, turkey, fish, or lean beef) and as many vegetables as you can fit on your plate. If there is a starchy side dish that appeals to you, then take a sensible serving. Take one or two bites of the things you really crave—the first bite tastes best, anyway—and concentrate on savoring the food. You will tend to eat less and enjoy it much more.

You can eat any holiday food you want as long as you hold yourself accountable in your food journal and the portion sizes remain in keeping with your eating plan. Knowing that no food is off-limits will allow you to indulge without feeling that you have completely blown your diet and therefore might as well go on an all-out binge.

## What to Do When You Have a Strong Craving for a Sweet Treat

A little bit of sugar is fine, but most processed sweets—the ones that give the biggest sugar fix—have no redeeming nutritional value and leave you feeling lethargic once the initial high wears off.

Fresh fruit is a great choice because it is not just sweet but filled with fiber to keep you feeling full. Dried fruit is another good option because its sweetness rivals candy. But be careful with portion size—although dried fruit is chockful of vitamins and fiber, it also packs as much as four times the sugar and calories per ounce as its fresh counterparts. Choose dried fruits that are 100 percent natural with no sugar added and limit dried fruits that are sweetened with fruit juice and other sugars, which add excess calories. Dried apples, figs, raisins, apricots, and prunes often contain no added sugar. Dried cranberries, dried pineapple, and banana chips are among the dried fruit that are often processed with sugar or fruit juice to increase sweetness. The best way to determine if sugar has been added is to look at the label and ingredient list. Avoid words like "glacé" and "naturally sweetened," and any fruits where sugar or fruit juice are among the first three ingredients listed on the ingredient list.

Whole-grain crackers with low-fat cream cheese and a tablespoon of jam, nonfat frozen yogurt topped with All-Bran Bran Buds, sugar-free hot cocoa, a Tofutti Chocolate Fudge Treat or sugar-free Fudgsicle, and even a nonfat cappuccino sweetened with Truvia are all sweet treats that won't sabotage your diet.

If nothing but chocolate will do, take comfort in the fact that weight loss and chocolate don't have to be exclusive. Virtually every brand comes in a downsized version like Snickers miniatures, Reese's mini peanut butter cups, York Peppermint Patty mini, and Butterfinger's BB's. These mini versions of your favorite chocolate treats allow you to indulge your craving—once in a while—without going overboard.

## Staying on Track When You're Eating with Nondieters

Nothing erodes self-control like a friendly get-together. Dinner with friends, family barbecues, and ballpark outings are just a few of the social situations that can dissolve your best intentions to stick to your diet. Research has shown that people tend to overeat whenever they are in the company of others, especially family and friends. It's twice as difficult to show restraint when everyone around you is digging in and enjoying each tasty bite. We tend to forgive ourselves for eating poorly if everyone around us is doing the same. You've seen the trend: If one person orders dessert, everyone orders dessert.

What to do? First of all, when everyone is ordering fattening appetizers like buffalo wings or fried calamari, the worst thing you can do is order nothing. While everyone else is digging in, you'll be sitting there with nothing to eat. I recommend my clients always order a salad or a cup of soup to start a meal. Salad and soup are nutritious, low-calorie fare (especially if the dressing is on the side and the soup is creamless). These foods help to fill you up so you eat less of your entrée. In addition, busying yourself with your own first-course food will help you to avoid picking at your neighbor's more fattening appetizer.

The same theory applies to dessert. When everyone else is ordering ice cream and cake, and the waiter asks for your order, order something! Fresh fruit, hot tea, or skim-milk cappuccinos are all good options. And if you simply can't resist the fudge sundae next to you, then ask for an extra spoon and take just a bite or two. It certainly is better than eating an entire dessert of your own.

From day one on the F-Factor Diet, you can dine out at any restaurant, so ordering from the menu will not be a problem. For example, when I go with friends to an Italian restaurant, I order dishes I love like a chopped salad topped with a shaving of Parmesan cheese, grilled calamari, and zuppa di pesce (seafood in a tomato broth). I leave dinner full and satisfied without feeling like I missed out or blew my intentions to eat well.

Try to remember that the point of eating together is to spend quality time with your friends and family. The focus should be more on the conversation and less on the food. Let your loved ones know that you're serious about changing your eating habits, and encourage them to offer their support and understanding to help keep you on track.

## Frequently Asked Questions on Step 3

QUESTION: We eat at fast-food restaurants because our kids love it and it's inexpensive. How can I eat with them without falling off my diet?

ANSWER: Obesity is a growing epidemic, not just among American adults but among children as well. The entire family will benefit from cutting back on fast-food meals. But for those times when fast food is the only option, you can eat with your family without going off the program.

Choose salads and grilled foods instead of fried foods, which are high in fat and calories. Ask for toppings to be served on the side, especially the high-fat, high-calorie variety, like full-fat mayonnaise and salad dressings.

Eating French fries and other fried food once in a while, as a special treat, is fine—but try to split an order with a friend or order a small portion. In small amounts, these foods can still be part of a healthy diet.

QUESTION: Is it true that eating after 8:00 P.M. causes weight gain? Sometimes I work late and can't sit down for dinner before then. What should I do?

ANSWER: It doesn't matter what time of day you eat; it's how much you eat during the whole day and how much exercise you get that makes you gain or lose weight. No matter when you eat your meals, your body will store extra calories as fat. So if you come home after 8:00 P.M., you should still eat dinner. Aim for a meal of protein and vegetables rather than a meal heavy in carbohydrates.

If you want to have a snack before bedtime, make sure that you first think about how many servings of carbohydrates you have already eaten that day, and build your snack around that. Try not to snack while doing other things like watching television, playing video games, or using the computer. If you eat meals and snacks in the kitchen or dining room, you are less likely to be distracted and more likely to be aware of what and how much you are eating. If you do want to snack while watching TV, take a small amount of food with you—not the whole bag.

QUESTION: What do I do if I have a really bad day of eating? How do I get back on the program?

ANSWER: The important thing to remember is that losing weight is not a sprint but rather a marathon. When you look at your eating habits as a way of life rather than a quick, short-term solution to drop a few pounds, you realize that one bad day is not going to destroy your goal of losing weight and living healthfully. In fact, one bad day is just that—one bad day. In the big picture, it is just a blip on the screen.

I tell my clients that they should aim to eat well 90 percent of the time. Ten percent of the time, they are allowed some indulgent days. There are 365 days a year. If you take 10 percent of that, you get 36.5 days of not having to eat perfectly well. Does that mean that you can follow the plan all week and splurge every weekend? The answer is no. If you splurged every Saturday, that would be 52 days a year that you indulged—practically 15 more days than you are entitled to. And if you indulged all weekend, both Saturday and Sunday, now you are talking about 104 days of splurging—67 days more than I recommend!

So what does the 10 percent (36.5 days) cover? In essence, it allows you to enjoy life's celebrations while maintaining a healthy foundation. Often, these times are accompanied by delicious foods that, if not present, would make these occasions somehow incomplete. For example, what would your birthday be without a slice of birthday cake? Or how about Valentine's Day without a piece of chocolate? And what kind of Thanksgiving would it be without stuffing and pumpkin pie?

Holidays and celebrations are special times that mark our lives. I never want to see someone "dieting" on a holiday or on a vacation. I am not giving you carte blanche for a full-out binge but rather license for an indulgence every now and then. Because in fact, little indulgences make life special.

Life is short and I want you to enjoy it. Eating healthfully does not have to mean depriving yourself all the time. Actually, the 10 percent (36.5 days) allows you to enjoy special occasions without feelings of guilt. By returning the next day to the healthful eating habits you learned on the F-Factor Diet, you can maintain a healthy weight while enjoying life to the fullest.

## STEP 3 JOURNAL

| Date: | | Carb | Fiber |
|---|---|---|---|
| **BREAKFAST** | | | |
| | | | |
| | | | |
| | | | |
| | | | |
| **LUNCH** | | | |
| | | | |
| | | | |
| | | | |
| | | | |
| | | | |
| **SNACK** | | | |
| | | | |
| | | | |
| **DINNER/SUPPER** | | | |
| | | | |
| | | | |
| | | | |
| | | | |
| | | | |
| **SNACK/DESSERT** | | | |
| | | | |
| | | | |

$$A - B = C$$

$$g - g = g$$

ingested carb    fiber

<125 g net carb/day

| | g | g |
|---|---|---|
| | A | B >35 g |

## DINING OUT AND ORDERING IN

*I've known what it is to be hungry, but I always went right to a restaurant.*

—RING LARDNER

ACCORDING TO the National Restaurant Association, more than half of all adults eat in or carry out food from a restaurant every day. No longer just for special occasions, dining on restaurant fare has become an integral part of everyday life for convenience, variety, and taste.

Dining out doesn't need to sabotage a healthy lifestyle. In fact, the F-Factor Diet was initially devised to suit the hectic lives of my Manhattan clients, who work hard and play hard, with little time for preparing a home-cooked meal. The diet was created with the understanding that many people eat out at least two meals a day. Perhaps you eat breakfast on the way to work, lunch and an afternoon snack at your desk, and dinners for the most part at home. Or maybe breakfast is the only meal you eat in your own kitchen, often lunching and dining in restaurants.

If you like to cook and prepare your own meals, the recipes in Chapter 11 will come in handy. But if you are someone who uses the oven to store extra pairs of shoes, you'll find this chapter's tips for dining out and ordering in invaluable.

From day one of the F-Factor Diet, you can dine out without sabotaging your efforts to lose weight. Whether you choose Italian, French, Indian, Chinese, or Mexican cuisine, or stick to good old American fare, you will find plenty of options on the menu that fit into all three steps of the F-Factor Diet.

For example, on Step 1 when you focus on vegetables and lean proteins, a Chinese dinner may begin with soup, followed by a chicken stir-fry with vegetables. On Step 2, when you can incorporate three servings of high-fiber carbohydrates, that same Chinese dinner you had on Step 1 could include ⅔ cup of brown rice. And finally on Step 3, the maintenance phase, you can eat virtually any food in moderation.

Freedom to enjoy dining out without "blowing" your diet is finally here.

## Italian Food

Thanks to low-carb diets, pasta has undeservedly gotten a bad rap. We Americans were told that in order to lose weight we had to cut out carbohydrates like pasta, bread, and rice. Yet in Italy, where many people eat pasta every day in some regions, they do not have the incidence of obesity that we do in America. In Italy, pasta is never a main course, just a small first course (primo piatto).

A main course of spaghetti in the United States can have as much as 1,000 calories—that's more than half your total calories for the day. Instead of a main course pasta, opt for an appetizer portion that typically has as few as 300 calories. Follow your appetizer portion of pasta with an entrée of grilled fish or meat with a side of vegetables, and you have a delicious and satisfying meal. So don't be afraid to order pasta, just do it the way Italians do.

Authentic Italian meals always include vegetables. I recommend beginning your meal with a vegetable soup, salad, or grilled vegetable antipasto. Vegetables are packed with fiber and fill you up for few calories. Starting a meal with a vegetable-based appetizer will enable you to eat less of your entrée while remaining full and satisfied. I also recommend ordering cooked vegetables (spinach, broccoli, or string beans) as a side dish to your entrée. Just make sure to avoid oil-laden vegetable dishes like fried zucchini and eggplant Par-

migiana, which contain excess fat and calories. Eggplant Parmigiana, which is breaded, fried, and topped with mozzarella cheese, tips the scales at 1,200 calories a serving. Opt for grilled eggplant in tomato sauce instead. You'll get an added bonus: tomato sauce contains lycopene, a cancer-fighting phyto-chemical.

Chicken cacciatore, zuppa di pesce (a seafood stew in a tomato broth), and grilled calamari (not fried!) are all good choices. Skip the breadbasket and tiramisù and have a glass of red wine and a low-fat cappuccino for dessert instead.

ITALIAN HEALTHY CHOICES
red or white wine
roasted peppers
marinated mushrooms
minestrone soup
tricolor salad
seafood salad
grilled calamari
steamed clams or mussels
pasta with marinara sauce
pasta Bolognese
pasta primavera with
    tomato-based sauce
pasta with clam sauce (red or white)
zuppa di pesce (seafood in a
    red sauce)
grilled fish
chicken marsala
chicken cacciatore
veal or chicken piccata
vegetable pizza (whole-wheat, thin
    crust is healthiest)

Italian ice
fresh fruit
cappuccino (made with skim
    or low-fat milk)

ITALIAN FOODS TO AVOID
fried mozzarella
fried calamari
garlic bread, Italian bread
Caesar salad
sausage, meatballs, or pepperoni
    in heroes, on pizza
lasagna
baked ziti
manicotti
fettuccine Alfredo
pasta carbonara
shrimp scampi
veal or chicken scaloppine
veal, chicken or eggplant
    Parmigiana
cannoli, spumoni, and tartufo

Sample meal for dining in an Italian restaurant during Step 1:
* tricolor salad with shaved Parmesan and aged balsamic vinegar

- zuppa di pesce or grilled veal chops Milanese (with chopped arugula and tomatoes)
- 1 serving of strawberries

TOTAL Carbohydrate: 15 grams     TOTAL Fiber: 10 grams

Sample meal for dining in an Italian restaurant during Step 2:
- appetizer pasta primavera (1½ cups pasta with vegetables) with 1 tablespoon of Parmesan cheese
- zuppa di pesce (mixed seafood in a light tomato broth)
- 1 glass red wine

TOTAL Carbohydrate: 15 grams     TOTAL Fiber: 10 grams

## Chinese Food

In China, cooking generally emphasizes large amounts of grains and vegetables and limited portions of meat, which is consistent with healthy eating. Unfortunately, Chinese food in the United States caters to Americans' taste for fried foods and meat-based entrées rather than vegetables and grains.

When choosing entrées in a Chinese restaurant, aim for low-fat choices like stir-fried or steamed dishes loaded with vegetables and lean protein such as chicken and seafood. If steamed entrées are too bland for your palate, order one stir-fried selection and one steamed selection and mix the two together to share. The abundant sauce will flavor both and reduce the calorie and fat content of the stir-fried choice. For an additional savings, always ask that your stir-fried dishes be prepared with minimal oil. For every tablespoon of oil omitted, you save 120 calories and 14 grams of fat. Most Chinese restaurants will happily oblige, and I promise you won't taste the difference.

Limit your intake of fatty spareribs, fried wontons, egg rolls, shrimp toast, and fried rice (loaded with oil). Anything labeled "sweet and sour" invariably means fried and coated in a sugary sauce. Steer away from other fried entrées such as General Tso's chicken, crispy orange beef, and kung pao chicken. Kung pao chicken can contain a cup of cashews and 1,275 calories, and it has the same amount of fat as four McDonald's Quarter Pounders. A better choice would be sautéed chicken with broccoli, a low-fat dish with only 250 calories.

White rice is a staple in Chinese restaurants. While it contains no fat, white rice also contains virtually no fiber. The good news is that because of popular demand, many Chinese restaurants now offer brown rice, which has more nutrients than white rice, and contains 6 grams of fiber per cup.

To limit sodium, ask that your food be prepared without salt or MSG, and request that soy sauce be served on the side.

CHINESE HEALTHY CHOICES

wonton soup
hot and sour soup
steamed dumplings
chicken, seafood, beef, or tofu and
    vegetables—stir-fried or steamed
steamed fish
moo-shu vegetables, shrimp,
    or chicken
steamed brown rice
soy, duck, and plum sauce
fortune cookies

CHINESE FOODS TO AVOID

egg drop soup
fried wontons
egg rolls
fried dumplings
spareribs
house fried rice
house lo mein
egg foo yung
noodles with sesame sauce
cashew chicken
lemon/orange chicken (if fried)
sesame chicken
General Tso's chicken
orange (crispy) beef
sweet-and-sour pork
lobster sauce

Sample meal for dining in a Chinese restaurant during Step 1:
- 1 cup tofu vegetable soup
- grilled beef satay (with sauce on side)
- sautéed scallops and shrimp with broccoli in garlic sauce

TOTAL Carbohydrate: 0 grams    TOTAL Fiber: 9 grams

Sample meal for dining in a Chinese restaurant during Step 2:
- hot and sour soup
- happy family (sliced beef, chicken, jumbo shrimp with broccoli, water chestnut, and bell pepper)
- ⅓ cup brown rice

TOTAL Carbohydrate: 20 grams    TOTAL Fiber: 9 grams

# French Food

Sauces are the heart of classic French food or haute cuisine, with good reason, but they are often filled with artery-clogging fat that goes straight to your heart. White sauces and béchamel often contain cream, while hollandaise and béarnaise are cholesterol heavyweights containing egg yolks and butter. Break tradition and ask for these sauces on the side, or opt for more healthy alternatives, such as bordelaise and other sauces with a wine base. Avoid creamy, cheesy dishes (anything au gratin) and high-fat meat dishes like pâté and foie gras.

Newer French cuisine or "nouvelle" is often prepared with healthier ingredients and cooking methods. A good rule for French dining is to keep it simple. Steamed mussels or salad, with dressing on the side, are good ways to begin a meal. Grilled meats and fish are healthy choices for entrées. Bouillabaisse is a traditional French dish made from seafood in a light tomato broth and is low in fat. Niçoise salad, a large salad with tuna, eggs, string beans, and greens, is another great choice. To make it even lighter, ask for the dressing on the side and omit the potatoes.

The good news with French food is portion size. The French don't supersize the way we do—they enjoy quality over quantity. Rich foods in small portions make for controlled decadence.

FRENCH HEALTHY CHOICES
red or white wine
consommé
whole-wheat baguettes
endive, watercress, or Niçoise salad
saumon fumé d'Écosse
    (Scottish smoked salmon)
tuna tartare
moules marinières (mussels
    steamed in shallots and
    white wine)
poached or steamed fish
whole roasted fish

chicken in wine sauce
rotisserie chicken
grilled steak (l'onglet à l'échalote,
    faux-filet Bercy)
duck breast (remove the skin)
fresh, poached, flambéed, or wine-
    soaked fruit

FRENCH FOODS TO AVOID
quiche
croissants
baguettes made with white flour
cream-based or cheese-topped soups

pâté
foie gras
cheese fondue
côte de boeuf (prime rib)
gratin de macaroni (penne pasta,
   Parisian ham and Gruyère)

pommes frites (French fries)
béarnaise, hollandaise, béchamel or
   mornay sauce
au gratin
pastries and éclairs
brioche

Sample meal for dining in a French restaurant during Step 1:
* French onion soup (no bread or cheese)
* mesclun à l'huile d'olive (mesclun salad and olive oil vinaigrette)
* moules marinières (fresh mussels cooked in a light shallot and white wine sauce)

TOTAL Carbohydrate: 0 grams     TOTAL Fiber: 3 grams

Sample meal for dining in a French restaurant during Step 2:
* thon tartare (tuna tartare)
* l'onglet (hanger steak with black pepper sauce, on the side)
* steamed asparagus
* glass of red wine

TOTAL Carbohydrate: 15 grams     TOTAL Fiber: 5 grams

## Japanese Food

Today, sushi bars are the fastest-growing restaurant segment of the ethnic food industry. That's good news for Americans, because if you're in search of a healthy meal, Japanese food fits the bill. Traditional Japanese food is most often prepared with little oil and features ingredients like tofu, rice, seaweed, noodles, vegetables, and small quantities of fish, chicken, and lean meat. Most sauces are low-fat, made with a base of broth, soy sauce, or sake.

For the lightest appetizers, go for flavorful miso soup (50 calories), a house green salad with ginger dressing (110 calories), or a seaweed salad (110 calories). Edamame (steamed soy beans) are high in fiber, protein, and isoflavones. Skip the fried pork dumplings and opt for steamed shrimp dumplings instead for a savings of 100 calories.

Sashimi (raw fish) and sushi (vinegared rice prepared with seaweed, raw fish, and/or vegetables) are good low-fat, high-protein choices. Many sushi bars will even prepare your sushi with brown rice if they have it. Sushi and sashimi are also excellent sources of omega-3 fatty acids, heart-healthy fats that may reduce the risk of cardiovascular disease. Stick with lean fish like tuna, crab, shrimp, snapper, scallop, and fluke and go easy on higher-fat fishes such as yellowtail, salmon, and eel. Sashimi is a great option for Step 1 of the program since it has no rice. And with each slice of fish averaging only 15 calories, you can get a lot of bang for your buck.

If you are a sushi beginner, ask which types of fish are cooked—not all sushi is raw. Crab, shrimp, eel, and salmon are often cooked, and sushi rolls can be made with just vegetables if you prefer.

As sushi becomes more and more mainstream, many rolls are being created to suit the high-fat palate of American diners. Avoid rolls such as spider rolls (fried soft-shell crab) and shrimp tempura rolls prepared with fried ingredients, and rolls prepared with high-fat ingredients like the New York roll (smoked salmon and cream cheese).

If you don't like sushi, there are many healthy cooked foods to choose from. Good choices include: chicken, salmon, or beef teriyaki, chicken sukiyaki

Eating raw or undercooked fish or shellfish does carry some risk. Children, pregnant women, and people with liver disorders or weakened immune systems are particularly vulnerable to getting sick. Foods made with raw fish are more likely to contain parasites such as tapeworms, flatworms, and roundworms. Luckily, the National Academy of Sciences has found that human parasitic infections from seafood are rare in the United States, and as yet there is no evidence of a significant increase due to the growing popularity of raw fish dishes. The FDA also recently reviewed seafood safety issues and concluded that the vast majority of seafood in the marketplace is safe to eat, and overall, American shoppers can be confident that the fish they buy will provide a healthful meal. A recent FDA study estimated that the risk of illness from seafood was one illness per 250,000 servings. The same study estimated a risk of about one illness in every 25,000 servings of chicken. If you are concerned about parasites in fish and seafood, order them fully cooked to reduce the risk.

(a one-pot dish of chicken, tofu, bamboo shoots, and vegetables simmered in broth at your table) and shabu-shabu (sliced beef and vegetables with noodles, cooked and served at the table).

What to avoid? Anything tempura, which is battered and deep-fried. Just 4 pieces of shrimp tempura can rack up 800 calories. Do you think vegetable tempura is a healthy option? Think again. Even vegetable tempura contains about 600 calories per serving.

Last, go easy on soy and teriyaki sauces as well as on miso dressing. Although they are virtually fat-free, they contain a lot of sodium, which can make you feel bloated. Get these sauces on the side whenever possible, ask for a smaller amount, and ask if low-sodium sauces are available.

JAPANESE HEALTHY CHOICES
Miso soup
seaweed salad
mixed salad with ginger dressing
sashimi salad
tuna tataki
edamame
steamed shumai (shrimp dumpling)
sushi pieces and rolls
sashimi (raw fish, no rice)
naruto roll (fish wrapped in cucumber, no rice)
steamed vegetable dishes
oshitashi (boiled spinach)
yakitori (chicken breast on skewers)
grilled Chilean sea bass, salmon, shrimp
nabemono (casserole)
yosenabe (seafood and vegetables in broth)

shabu-shabu (beef with vegetables and noodles)
sumashi wan (tofu and shrimp in broth)
chicken, fish, or beef teriyaki
low-sodium soy sauce

JAPANESE FOODS TO AVOID
vegetable, chicken, or seafood tempura
tempura roll
tonkatsu (breaded pork)
fried dumplings
fried bean curd
oyako domburi (chicken and eggs over rice)
chawan mush (egg custard with chicken and shrimp)
yo kan (bean cake)
regular soy sauce

Sample meal for dining in a Japanese restaurant during Step 1:
• green salad with ginger dressing

- miso soup
- sashimi dinner: 3 pieces tuna, 3 pieces yellowtail, 3 pieces salmon, 3 pieces shrimp
- green tea

TOTAL Carbohydrate: 0 grams      TOTAL Fiber: 3 grams

Sample meal for dining in a Japanese restaurant during Step 2:
- seaweed salad
- chicken yakitori (2 skewers)
- tuna and scallion roll
- 1 California roll

TOTAL Carbohydrate: 45 grams      TOTAL Fiber: 4 grams

## Mexican Food

When you sit down for Mexican food, one thing is certain: the ubiquitous bowl of free nacho chips awaits you at your table. As you read the menu, deciding what to order, it is only natural that you dig in and crunch away. But watch out. For every 15 chips, you take in 200 calories. And every time you dip a chip in guacamole, you're adding another 35 calories. Do the math: 15 chips with guacamole adds up to 675 calories—and that is before you have had a bite of your entrée! Instead, ask your server to remove the chips and replace them with corn tortillas (80 calories) or whole-wheat tortillas (100 calories) and salsa.

Keep your appetizer light by ordering black bean or tortilla soup—both are flavorful and filling and have less than 200 calories for a cup. The black bean soup also gives you the added benefit of 8 grams of filling fiber. What to avoid? Nachos grande (with beef, guacamole, and sour cream), which can easily contain 1,400 calories per serving. Even an innocent quesadilla racks up 500 calories.

The best entrées are those that are grilled and contain vegetables and protein. Fajitas, prepared with chicken, shrimp, or lean beef, are healthy and delicious choices. Use the peppers and onions to fill the soft tortillas instead of sour cream, cheese, and guacamole. Other good choices include a vegetable or chicken burrito and soft chicken tacos. Ask your waiter to prepare these dishes with whole-wheat tortillas for a fiber boost.

Avoid the beef chimichanga, a deep-fried flour tortilla stuffed with meat and cheese. It will set you back 800 calories. Enchiladas and quesadillas mostly consist of white-flour tortillas stuffed with some combination of rice, beans, cheese, and beef or chicken, and arrive loaded with fat and calories.

While beans are a great source of lean protein and fiber, refried beans are a different story. Refried beans are just that: beans fried in lard, often with added bacon or cheese. No wonder a ¾-cup serving has a third of a day's worth of saturated fat. Instead, order a side of black beans and rice.

The good news is that more and more Mexican restaurants are now advertising "healthy" Mexican food. They no longer use lard in cooking; they use lean cuts of meat, and they offer more vegetarian dishes. If you avoid dishes full of cheese and don't partake in a large bowl of guacamole with chips, you don't have to say "adios" to Mexican food.

MEXICAN HEALTHY CHOICES
gazpacho
black bean soup
chicken, shrimp, or mixed vegetable
    fajitas
chicken vegetable enchiladas
    without cheese topping
arroz con pollo
entrées featuring grilled fish
    or chicken
frijoles a la charra
borracho beans and rice
soft chicken or fish tacos
burritos without cheese
ceviche
salsa and pico de gallo
whole-wheat tortillas

MEXICAN FOODS TO AVOID
tortilla chips
chili con queso dip
nachos
entrées with chorizo (sausage) or
    carne frita (fried beef)
refried beans (made with lard)
beef tacos
cheese or beef enchiladas
quesadillas
burritos with cheese
chimichangas
guacamole and sour cream
churros and sopaipillas (fried dough
    desserts)

Sample meal for dining in a Mexican restaurant during Step 1:
- gazpacho
- chicken fajitas with peppers, onions, and salsa (no tortilla)

TOTAL Carbohydrate: 0 grams      TOTAL Fiber: 5 grams

Sample meal for dining in a Mexican restaurant during Step 2:

- tossed salad with 2 slices of avocado
- soft fish taco (use 1 whole-wheat tortilla)
- ⅓ cup black beans
- 1 margarita on the rocks

TOTAL Carbohydrate: 45 grams     TOTAL Fiber: 8 grams

## Greek Food

Greek food is one of the healthiest cuisines in the world. Typical of the Mediterranean diet, it relies heavily on vegetables, plenty of fish, and monounsaturated fats such as olive oil and nuts.

For appetizers, begin with a Greek salad (limit feta cheese to no more than 2 ounces), a whole-wheat pita with a tablespoon each of hummus, tzatziki (a yogurt cucumber sauce) and baba ghanoush (a creamy eggplant dip), or grilled calamari. Heart-healthy and waist-friendly entrées are plentiful. Grilled fish and shellfish are low-fat, high-protein staples. Plaki—fish cooked with tomatoes, onions, and garlic—is a flavorful and light entrée. Kebabs—especially chicken—in which the meat is grilled on a skewer with tomato, onion, and peppers, are also good low-fat, high-protein choices.

For the most part, it's hard to go wrong at a Greek restaurant. But there are a few dishes that are diet disasters: moussaka (baked eggplant, chopped meat, béchamel, and fresh herbs) and pastitsio (pasta casserole with spiced ground lamb topped with béchamel). Both dishes contain a rich cream sauce, which adds lots of fat and calories. Also, be careful of dishes prepared with phyllo dough. Although phyllo is flaky and feels light, the many layers are brushed with butter to make them crispy. Dishes such as spinach pie (spanakopita) and baklava are deceptively high in calories and fat. To limit the amount of sodium in a Greek meal, eat olives, anchovies, and feta cheese in moderation.

GREEK HEALTHY CHOICES

tzatziki (yogurt, garlic, and cucumber)

hummus (sesame paste and chickpeas)

baba ghanoush (eggplant, tahini, and olive oil)

tabouli

whole-wheat pita

seafood salad

house salad

Greek salad (limit feta cheese to 1–2 oz)

tomato salad

torato soup (cold soup made with eggplant, peppers, and yogurt)

horta (steamed greens with virgin olive oil and lemon dressing)

grilled calamari (squid)

grilled octopus

grilled portobello mushrooms

gigantes (butter beans baked in tomato sauce, herbs, and olive oil)

grilled fish (halibut, tuna, sole, snapper, swordfish, tilapia, loup de mer, salmon, sea bass, shrimp, scallops)

fish in plaki sauce (broiled with tomato and garlic)

kebabs (chicken, beef, lamb, shrimp)

lamb youvetsi (baked in a clay pot with orzo—or pasta—and tomato)

souvlaki (grilled lamb)

Greek yogurt with fresh fruit

GREEK FOODS TO AVOID

fried calamari

fried zucchini

spinach pie

country-style sausage

haloumi cheese (grilled cheese)

grape leaves (*dolmades*)

taramasalata (caviar mousse)

white pita bread

moussaka

pastitsio

baklava

loukoumades (fritters drizzled with honey)

Sample meal for dining in a Greek restaurant during Step 1:
- Greek salad with 2 oz of feta cheese
- lamb shish kebab
- horta

TOTAL Carbohydrate: 15 grams     TOTAL Fiber: 10 grams

Sample meal for dining in a Greek restaurant during Step 2:
- ½ whole-wheat pita with 1 tbsp. hummus and 1 tbsp. baba ghanoush
- ½ cup gigantes
- snapper in plaki sauce

TOTAL Carbohydrate: 45 grams     TOTAL Fiber: 15 grams

# Indian Food

Indian cuisine is often considered a prime example of a heart-healthy, plant-based diet. Traditional Indian dishes feature a variety of vegetables, beans, rice, lentils, and chickpeas—all of which provide carbohydrates and fiber. Indian cuisine relies heavily on spices that add flavor without adding fat: curries, black pepper, cinnamon, cloves, tamarind, chili, and cumin. Excellent choices include tandoori dishes like chicken, meat, or fish, which are marinated and oven-baked and are low in fat. Chicken or beef tikka (grilled) and chicken saag (with spinach) are other healthful choices. Tomato-based side dishes with beans or chickpeas, and vegetables in light sauces are a great accompaniment. And while I always recommend brown rice over white, Indian basmati rice is an exception. Although white in appearance, basmati rice is higher in protein and fiber than traditional white rice, so enjoy!

While Indian food can be healthy, there are some trouble spots to avoid. Watch out for dishes that have large amounts of ghee (clarified butter) poured on top for flavor. Items that include the words "kandhari," "malai," or "kurma" indicate dishes high in cream and coconut milk. Some curries are made with large amounts of coconut milk and cream as well, so be sure to ask your restaurant server how the food is prepared; lighter oils are often available on request. Curries can be made with a yogurt-based sauce instead of a coconut milk, so don't hesitate to ask.

All Indian meals are accompanied by fresh bread. Avoid deep-fried poori, samosas (fried meat or vegetable turnovers), and pakori (deep-fried breads and vegetables). Choose baked breads such as whole-wheat chapati and naan instead.

INDIAN HEALTHY CHOICES
tamata salat (tomato salad)
mulligatawny soup
    (lentils and vegetables)
chicken or beef tikka
tandoori chicken, fish, or beef
chicken, fish, or beef saag
    (spinach)

chicken, fish, or beef vindaloo
    (potatoes and leeks)
shish kebab
gobhi matar tamata (cauliflower with
    peas and tomatoes)
matar pulao (rice with peas)
papadum or papad
    (lentil wafers)

whole-wheat naan or chapati
basmati rice

INDIAN FOODS TO AVOID
anything made with coconut milk
   or cream (soup, curries, etc.)

fried breads
pakora (fried dough with vegetables)
samosas (fried vegetable turnovers)
chicken masala
saag paneer (spinach in cream)
white naan

Sample meal for dining in an Indian restaurant during Step 1:
- tamata salat
- chicken tikka
- gobhi matar

TOTAL Carbohydrate: 0 grams    TOTAL Fiber: 5 grams

Sample meal for dining in an Indian restaurant during Step 2:
- 1 piece of whole-wheat chapati
- tandoori chicken
- ⅓ cup basmati rice
- 1 cup mulligatawny soup

TOTAL Carbohydrate: 30 grams    TOTAL Fiber: 10 grams

## Fast Food

America has been called a fast-food nation, and for good reason. Fast-food restaurants are growing at an overwhelming rate. Today, McDonald's has 14,157 locations; Pizza Hut has 7,756 locations; Dunkin' Donuts has 7,200 locations; Burger King has 7,183 locations; and the granddaddy of them all, Subway, has over 25,903 locations in the United States.

Every day, 1 out of 4 Americans eats fast food. Most do it for the convenience—lack of time leads many people to the drive-through. Money plays a part as well—if you are eating out, fast-food restaurants are often the cheapest option. But economics and time are not the only reasons Americans like fast food. Fast food caters to Americans' appetite for calorie-dense foods high in sodium and fat. Simply put, many Americans like the taste.

Unfortunately, much of the food offered in fast-food restaurants lacks important nutrients like fiber, vitamins, and minerals. Until recently, French fries were the only vegetable option at many fast-food restaurants.

As the epidemic of obesity grew into a national concern, many were quick to blame fast food as the cause of Americans' expanding waistlines. In response, fast-food establishments have been forced to create healthy alternatives. Arby's added a grilled chicken barbecue sandwich; Burger King removed half the fat from its BK broiler chicken sandwich and offers the MorningStar veggie burger; Subway offers a Fresh Fit Choices menu; and Wendy's added a grilled chicken sandwich and salads. Dairy Queen and Baskin-Robbins have introduced low-fat and nonfat frozen yogurt, and McDonald's introduced a fruit 'n yogurt parfait and individually packaged apple slices. Even Dunkin' Donuts eliminated egg yolks from doughnuts and introduced bagels to their menus.

Fresh fruit, salads, low-fat muffins, low-fat milk and yogurt, and grilled sandwiches are now fast-food menu staples. While nothing is more nutritious than a home-cooked meal, with all the healthier additions to the menus it is now possible to eat sensibly at a fast-food chain.

## Order It Your Way

What you choose to eat can greatly affect the nutritional quality of your meal. Your overall objectives are to reduce fat, calories, and sodium, and add fiber. Here are some specific tactics to employ:

- Eliminate high-fat sauces and dressings, or order on the side and use sparingly:
  - mayonnaise (2 tbsp. = 194 calories, 21 g fat)
  - tartar sauce (134 calories, 14 g fat, per serving)
  - cheese (processed American, 100 calories, 7 g fat, per slice)
  - salad dressing (2 oz olive oil and vinegar = 310 calories, 33 g fat)

- Choose grilled or broiled version of foods, rather than fried alternatives.
- When ordering pizza, opt for vegetable toppings and a thin crust. Ask for whole-wheat crust for extra fiber.
- Whenever possible, order a salad, and fill up on vegetables, fruit, and beans.
- Go easy on processed meats like bacon, pepperoni, and sausage, which are high in fat, sodium, and carcinogenic nitrates.
- Choose low-fat muffins, cereal, and low-fat milk for breakfast foods, while avoiding biscuits (235 calories, 12 g fat) and croissants (180 calories, 10 g fat).

- Try the leaner beef versions of your favorite sandwich.
- Avoid super-sizing and value meals (more value actually equals more fat and calories).
- Remove skin from fried chicken (a major reservoir of fat) and fill out your meal with corn on the cob, baked potato, and salad.
- Order whole-grain versions of bread whenever available.
- Use baked potatoes as a side dish without elaborate toppings.
- Reduce calories by choosing juice or low-fat milk instead of soft drinks (310 calories for a large) or milk shakes (10 oz = 300–400 calories).

FAST-FOOD HEALTHY CHOICES

bagel with jelly and low-fat cream cheese

low-fat bran muffin

cereal with skim or low-fat milk

green salads with light dressing

plain hamburgers (small size)

grilled chicken sandwiches (no sauce)

turkey burgers

veggie burgers

lean roast beef or turkey subs (no mayo) on whole-wheat roll

entrée salads with grilled chicken or shrimp

baked potatoes topped with salsa or vegetarian chili

chili made with beans

ketchup, mustard, honey mustard, or barbecue sauce

fruit 'n yogurt parfait

low-fat frozen yogurt

apple slices with dipping sauce

low-fat milk

bottled water

FAST-FOOD ITEMS TO AVOID

biscuits

danish

doughnuts

croissant breakfast sandwiches (and croissants or pastries in general)

egg sandwiches, especially those with sausage or bacon

hash browns

burgers with cheese, "special sauce," and/or mayonnaise

fried chicken or fried fish fillet sandwiches

chicken nuggets

fried chicken

mashed potatoes

large and jumbo-size French fries

baked potatoes with butter, sour cream, or cheese

nachos

onion rings

soft drinks

milk shakes

Sample meal for dining at McDonald's during Step 1:
- Bacon Ranch Grilled Chicken Salad (no cheese) with Newman's Own Low-Fat Balsamic Vinaigrette Dressing
- medium iced tea (unsweetened)

TOTAL Carbohydrate: 20 grams     TOTAL Fiber: 3 grams

Sample meal for dining at McDonald's during Step 2:
- side salad with Newman's Own Low-Fat Balsamic Vinaigrette Dressing
- Artisan Grilled Chicken Sandwich
- medium Diet Coke

TOTAL Carbohydrate: 47 grams     TOTAL Fiber: 4 grams

The most important thing to remember when eating out is to think of it as part of your overall healthy eating plan. Try to order wisely. And, if portions are big or the food is rich, consider taking some of it home for a meal the next day. Also, consider sharing entrées, appetizers, or desserts with dining partners. Moderation is always key, but planning ahead can help you relax and enjoy your dining-out experience without sacrificing good nutrition or diet control.

With just a little thought and awareness, you can make healthy choices in restaurants. No longer does being on a diet mean that you are stuck home preparing complicated meals every night. From day one on the F-Factor Diet, readers can enjoy dining out with friends and family while sticking to the program and losing weight.

CHAPTER

**10**

# EXERCISE TO EMPTY YOUR GLYCOGEN STORES

*The physically fit can enjoy their vices.*
—LORD PERCIVAL

No BOOK about weight loss can ignore the vital role exercise plays in burning calories, enhancing cardiovascular health, and—for the F-Factor Diet in particular—emptying your glycogen stores. There is no question: adding exercise to any diet program is the most efficient and healthiest way to lose weight.

The benefits of exercise are well known, and yet it's surprising how many people fail to do it. All of the advances of modern technology—from electric can openers to remote controls—have made life easier, more comfortable, and much less physically demanding. According to the CDC, more than 1 in 4 U.S. adults over 50 do not engage in regular physical activity. The number-one excuse people gave for not exercising is lack of time. Ironically, on average, Americans are watching five hours of television per day! To make matters worse, many of us snack mindlessly while watching television. Research shows that we automatically overdo portions when we snack in front of the television, especially when eating straight from the package.[19] Unfortunately, we're not snacking on carrot sticks or apples but rather on foods like chips, pretzels, cookies, and ice cream (foods low in fiber and high in calories). One thing is certain: Americans are eating more and moving less, and our waistlines are paying the price.

Combining the F-Factor Diet with exercise is the most powerful formula for losing body fat. Your body weight is determined by the amount of calories you take in and the amount of calories you burn: take in more calories than you burn and you will gain weight. The F-Factor Diet controls caloric intake by filling you up on lean protein and high-fiber foods; adding exercise burns excess calories that otherwise would be stored as fat.

During my years of practice, I have seen many patients try to diet without making exercise an integral component of their weight-loss efforts. And the results are always the same. While they may lose weight temporarily, keeping it off is almost impossible. By increasing your daily physical activity and decreasing your caloric input, you could lose excess weight in the most efficient and healthful way with a better chance at keeping it off.

**Exercise can:**

give you more stamina and energy

reduce stress and improve sleep

help you lose body fat and keep it off

increase strength by building muscle

reduce your risk of chronic disease such as heart disease and diabetes

lower high blood pressure

keep bones healthy at all ages

---

19. D. A. Redelmeier and M. B. Stanbrook, "Television Viewing and Risk of Obesity," *Journal of the American Medical Association* 290 (July 2003): 332. See also F. B. Hu, T. Y. Li, G. A. Colditz, et al., "Television Watching and Other Sedentary Behaviors in Relation to Risk of Obesity and Type 2 Diabetes Mellitus in Women," *Journal of the American Medical Association* 289 (April 2003): 1785–91.

# The Benefits of Exercising on the F-Factor Diet

## 1. Deplete Your Glycogen Stores

The carbohydrates you eat eventually end up as glucose to be stored as glycogen. Remember that the major portion of your glycogen is stored in your muscles. Only when these stores are full, and there is no more room for the glucose to be stored as glycogen, does your body convert and store the excess glucose as fat. Aside from limiting your intake of refined carbohydrates, the best way to keep those stores from overflowing is—yes—to exercise.

When you exercise, the energy that sustains you comes from your glycogen stores. The more you exercise, the more glycogen you use, therefore making more room for glucose to be stored later on. If there is enough room for the glucose in your muscles, there will be nothing left over to be stored as fat—and you are able to eat more carbohydrates without overflowing your stores. This explains how athletes can consume diets high in carbohydrates and remain slim and fit. Athletes often carbo-load (eat a lot of carbohydrates) before athletic events because they need glucose to sustain activity. For example, when you go for a long run, the energy comes from glycogen stored in your muscles. When a person does not exercise and eats excess refined carbohydrates (a lifestyle of most of the American population), his or her glycogen stores quickly reach capacity, and the spillover of glucose gets converted into fat.

## 2. Speed Up Your Metabolism

Research shows overwhelmingly that combining the proper diet with exercise is much more effective for losing body fat than dieting alone.[20] Dieting, or reducing your caloric intake, will result in dropping pounds, but keeping the weight off long term is almost impossible. Dieting without exercise results in weight cycling and is detrimental to your resting metabolic rate (RMR). RMR is the energy required to maintain vital body functions. The higher your RMR, the more calories you burn at rest and

---

20. C. J. Zelasko, "Exercise for Weight Loss: What Are the Facts?" *Journal of the American Dietetic Association* 95, no. 12 (December 1995): 1414–17. See also J. M. Rippe and S. Hesse, "The Role of Physical Activity in the Prevention and Management of Obesity," *Journal of the American Dietetic Association* 98, no. 10 (October 1998, supplement): S31–S38.

the less likely you are to gain weight. When the body perceives a reduction in caloric intake, it responds by conserving energy (decreasing RMR), therefore making it easier to regain weight.

Weight training has the added benefit of increasing an individual's RMR. The more muscle you have, the higher your RMR. Muscle is more metabolically active than fat, meaning it burns more calories. The more muscle you have, the greater your RMR and the more calories your body will burn. By incorporating even light weight training into your weekly workouts, you can change your body composition from fat to lean, and you will increase your RMR.

## 3. Improve Your Mental Health

The psychological benefits of exercise are equally important to the weight-conscious person. Exercise decreases stress and relieves tensions that might otherwise lead to overeating. When you exercise, hormones called endorphins are released, and endorphins give you a natural high and actually work to combat negative feelings.

Many people turn to food for comfort or a distraction from feelings of boredom, loneliness, anger, or frustration. For many, food provides a temporary comfort. The problem with this eating behavior is that while it may release stress in the short term, it creates more stress in the long term. For example, say you've had a rough day at work. Your boss criticized your work and belittled you in front of your colleagues. You return to your home exhausted, angry, and frustrated. You open the freezer and grab the pint of Ben & Jerry's. It is true that while you are eating, you may forget about the stresses of your day as you focus on how delicious the ice cream tastes. The problem is that eventually you will reach the end of the container. Once you are done eating, none of your troubles have gone away. And now, you have actually compounded the negative feelings with a new one: guilt. You feel guilty and disgusted with yourself for having binged. Turning to food for comfort creates a downward spiral of negativity.

What would be a healthier option? Hitting the gym, of course. When you exercise, the endorphins that get released actually work to combat negative feelings. I know that if I have had a bad day, going for an hour-long jog helps to clear my head, and I feel great when I'm done. After working out and doing something positive for myself, I actually *feel* more positive.

## 4. Regulate Appetite

Do you avoid exercise because you believe that it will just make you hungrier and lead to eating more? If so, you're not alone. Many people mistakenly think that exercise increases appetite to the point that extra food eaten will negate the number of calories burned. This is not the case. In fact, exercise may actually regulate your appetite, helping you to eat fewer calories than you would otherwise. Studies show that vigorous exercise increases body temperature.[21] The higher your body temperature, the more likely that your appetite will be suppressed for several hours following exercise.

There is also a strong psychological effect regulating food intake when you combine exercise with diet. Exercise builds physical fitness, which in turn builds self-confidence, enhanced self-image, and a positive outlook. When you start to feel good about yourself, you are more likely to want to make other positive changes in your lifestyle that will help keep your weight under control. People who regularly exercise typically eat a more healthy diet as well. After a great workout, you may think twice about returning home and ordering in a bucket of fried chicken.

It makes sense that if you commit your time and energy to do something healthy for yourself, you may think twice before sabotaging your goal by eating something fattening. When building the foundation of a true lifestyle change and commitment to health, diet and exercise work hand in hand.

## Getting Started

Pairing the F-Factor Diet with exercise results in the most weight loss in the shortest amount of time. If you already exercise regularly, keep up the good work. On the other hand, if you rarely work out, or maybe if you haven't worked out in years, now is the time to start. Begin with a basic walk around the neighborhood or even by mowing the lawn. The point is to get moving. The more you move, the more calories you burn. For beginners, 30 minutes

21. M. Gilliat-Wimberly, M. M. Manore, K. Woolf, et al., "Effects of Habitual Physical Activity on the Resting Metabolic Rates and Body Compositions of Women Aged 35 to 50 Years," *Journal of the American Dietetic Association* 101, no. 10 (October 2001): 1181–88.

of activity a few times a week is a great way to ease you into a workout routine. As time passes, your stamina and endurance will increase. Before you know it, you will be picking up the pace and feeling stronger and leaner every day.

You may be surprised at how many calories you can burn in just 1 hour, whether it is from a planned workout or just from housework. In the chart below, check the number closest to your weight to learn the approximate calorie burn for a variety of activities. The energy costs of activities that require you to move your own body weight, such as walking or jogging, are greater for heavier people since they have more weight to move. For example, a person weighing 190 pounds would burn more calories jogging 1 mile than a person jogging alongside who weighs 130 pounds. Always check to see what body weight is referred to in caloric expenditure charts you use.

| Physical Activities | Calories Burned in 1 Hour: 130 pounds | Calories Burned in 1 Hour: 155 pounds | Calories Burned in 1 Hour: 190 pounds |
|---|---|---|---|
| **GYM** | | | |
| aerobics, high impact | 413 | 493 | 604 |
| stationary bicycling, moderate pace | 413 | 493 | 604 |
| stationary bicycling, vigorously | 620 | 739 | 906 |
| boxing, punching bag | 708 | 844 | 1035 |
| elliptical trainer | 502 | 598 | 733 |
| stair-stepper machine | 354 | 422 | 518 |
| rowing machine | 413 | 493 | 604 |
| running 5 mph (12-min. mile) | 472 | 563 | 690 |
| running 8 mph (7.5-min. mile) | 797 | 950 | 1165 |
| walking, 4 mph, very brisk pace | 236 | 281 | 345 |
| weight lifting | 354 | 422 | 518 |
| **SPORTS & OUTDOORS** | | | |
| bicycling, 12–13.9 mph | 472 | 563 | 690 |
| dancing | 266 | 317 | 388 |
| Frisbee | 177 | 211 | 259 |
| golf, carrying clubs | 325 | 387 | 464 |
| hiking, cross-country | 354 | 422 | 518 |

| Physical Activities | Calories Burned in 1 Hour: 130 pounds | Calories Burned in 1 Hour: 155 pounds | Calories Burned in 1 Hour: 190 pounds |
|---|---|---|---|
| hockey, field & ice | 472 | 563 | 690 |
| horseback riding | 236 | 281 | 345 |
| skating, in-line | 413 | 493 | 604 |
| soccer, competitive | 413 | 493 | 604 |
| skiing, cross-country | 531 | 633 | 776 |
| tai chi | 236 | 281 | 345 |
| tennis | 472 | 563 | 690 |
| walking, 3.5 mph (17-min. mile) uphill | 354 | 422 | 518 |
| **HOME & DAILY LIFE** | | | |
| cleaning house, general | 207 | 246 | 302 |
| child care, bathing & feeding | 207 | 246 | 302 |
| cooking | 148 | 176 | 216 |
| food shopping, with cart | 177 | 211 | 259 |
| gardening | 295 | 352 | 431 |
| moving, carrying boxes | 413 | 493 | 604 |
| painting and remodeling | 266 | 317 | 388 |
| raking lawn | 236 | 272 | 345 |
| shoveling snow | 354 | 422 | 518 |

## Add Weight Training to Your Workouts

Adding weight training to your workouts produces numerous benefits. Like cardiovascular exercise, working out with weights burns calories during the actual workout. But unlike cardiovascular exercise, after an intense weight-training session your metabolism remains elevated hours after your workout has ended. In a recent study from the University of Colorado in Denver, women who did four sets of 10 exercises that targeted major body parts burned up to 60 extra calories in the hour right after lifting and kept burning at a higher level the rest of the day. This increase in metabolism results in your body burning more calories, even when doing nothing.

## Get the Most Out of Exercise

If you are working out to shed pounds, watching the clock is a smart move. Everyone agrees that you need to exercise. The debate continues about whether you receive the same benefits from three 10-minute bouts of aerobic exercise versus one 30-minute session. A recent study from Dalhousie University in Halifax, Nova Scotia, revealed that exercisers who walked for a half hour, 5 days a week for 8 weeks, significantly decreased their body fat, whereas those who did a trio of 10-minute stints throughout the day saw no marked body-fat change. It appears that your metabolism may stay fired up longer after a lengthy session, so you burn more calories.

The bottom line: If you are trying to lose weight, set aside at least 30 minutes of uninterrupted time for your workout.

---

Besides increasing metabolism, lifting weights makes you look leaner. Lifting weights increases your lean body mass. Fat does not "turn into" muscle, as is often believed. Fat and muscle are two entirely different substances and one cannot become the other. However, muscle does use calories at a faster rate than fat, which directly affects your body's metabolic rate or energy requirement. The more lean muscle you have, the higher your resting metabolic rate (RMR), and the more calories you burn each day while doing nothing.

Studies have estimated that for each pound of muscle that you add to your body, you burn another 35 to 50 calories per day. So an extra 10 pounds of muscle will burn approximately 350 to 500 calories a day, or an extra pound of fat every 7 to 10 days, without making any other changes.

Weight training is essential not only to losing body fat but also to keeping it off. By building up muscle during weight loss, you increase your metabolism instead of slowing it down. When you add muscle to your body, you greatly increase the number of calories you burn each day.

Once you achieve your goal weight, you can start eating more food without gaining back body fat, because of increased muscle mass and metabolism. More food without weight gain—brilliant! On the other hand, if you diet without lifting weights, you will lose fat *and* muscle. Losing muscle slows down your metabolism, leading to weight gain.

The benefits of exercise go beyond losing body fat. A fit body responds differently to things than a fat body. From a health standpoint, exercise positively affects every organ in your body. Exercise also improves your sleeping patterns, energy level, and overall feeling of well-being. The more you do, the more you will want to do as the benefits continue to increase and you get the results you're after. In short, exercise is a must for losing body fat as well as improving the overall quality of life. It will add years to your life and life to your years.

## Tips to Get You Started

By now, you should be convinced that in order to successfully manage your weight you must include exercise in your daily routine. Here are some tips to get you started:

- Check with your doctor first. If you are overweight and have other clinical conditions, it is wise to get your doctor's okay before embarking on an exercise program.
- Choose activities that you think you'll enjoy. Most people will stick to their exercise program if they are having fun, even though they are working hard.
- Set aside a regular exercise time. Whether this means joining an exercise class or getting up a little earlier every day, make time for this addition to your routine and don't let anything get in your way. Planning ahead will help you get around interruptions in your workout schedule, such as bad weather and vacations.
- Set short-term goals. Don't expect to lose 20 pounds in 2 weeks. It has taken a while for you to gain the weight; it will take time to lose it. Keep a record of your progress and tell your friends and family about your achievements.
- Vary your exercise program. Change exercises or invite friends to join you to make your workout more enjoyable. There is no "best" exercise—just the one that works best for you. It won't be easy, especially at the start. But as you begin to feel better, look better, and enjoy a new zest for life, you will be rewarded many times over for your efforts.

# THE F-FACTOR DIET IN PRACTICE

## THE F-FACTOR DIET RECIPES

*You don't have to cook fancy or complicated masterpieces—
just good food from fresh ingredients.*
—JULIA CHILD

THE F-FACTOR DIET differs from so many diets that require you to prepare special recipes in order to stick with the program.

From day one on the F-Factor Diet, you can follow the plan without cooking a thing: you can pour a bowl of cereal for breakfast, pick up lunch from a deli, and go out to any restaurant for dinner. The rationale for not needing to cook emerged because most of my New York City clients work hard and play hard. They do not have time to prepare home-cooked meals. And then there are those who do have the time, but simply do not like to cook. I had to create a program that was not dependent on a person's willingness to spend time in the kitchen.

On the other hand, for those of you who enjoy cooking, I have created over 80 recipes for you to prepare. One of the reasons I enjoy cooking is because I can control exactly what is going into my food: fresh, fiber-rich foods, lean proteins, and minimal amounts of added fat. When I cook, I can feel good about every bite that goes into my mouth.

The nutrition content for each recipe has been analyzed in two ways: 1) In keeping with the principles of the F-Factor Diet. Therefore, while the calorie and fiber contents are accurate, the carbohydrate contents have been reduced to reflect the zero grams of carbohydrate that the F-Factor Diet assigns to vegetables. Please use these for journaling. 2) The actual nutritional content includes the carbohydrate content of vegetables.

The recipes in this chapter are extremely simple, require few ingredients, and are easy to follow. Variety will keep your diet interesting. Lack of variety, on the other hand, will cause you to feel bored with your food choices and more likely one day to binge and stop following the program.

I hope that the simplicity of these recipes inspires you to get into the kitchen.

# STEP 1 RECIPES

## BREAKFAST FOODS

Berry Breakfast Parfait

Strawberry F-Factor Smoothie

F-Factor's Famous High-Fiber Pancakes

Greek Omelet

Apple Cinnamon "Oatmeal"

Heart-Healthy Turkey Sausage

## SOUP, SALADS, AND VEGETABLES

Chicken Soup

Vegetable Soup

Cabbage Soup

Grilled Sirloin Salad

Tuna-Egg Salad

Spinach Salad with Warm Bacon Vinaigrette

String Beans in Tomato Sauce

Broccoli Sesame Salad

Eggplant Rollatini

Blackened Green Beans

Roasted Brussels Sprouts

Cauliflower Pizza Crust

Sautéed Zucchini with Parmesan

Four Pepper Sauté

## CHICKEN AND TURKEY MAIN DISHES

Tandoori Chicken

Poached Chicken Salad with
    Raspberry Vinaigrette

Turkey Meat Loaf

Guiltless Chicken Parmesan

Southwest Turkey Burgers

## BEEF, PORK, AND LAMB MAIN DISHES

Classic Steak House Filet Mignon

TZ's Mozzarella-Stuffed Meatballs

Greek-Style Pork

Broiled Baby Lamb Chops

Grilled Veal Parmigiana

## FISH AND SHELLFISH MAIN DISHES

Shrimp with Feta Cheese

Crispy Tilapia

Broiled Salmon with Dill

Asian-Flavored Tuna

Maryland Crab Cakes

## SWEETS

Vanilla-Bean Applesauce

Macerated Fruit

Cheesecake Parfait with Blackberry Sauce

Grilled Fruit Kebabs

### BREAKFAST FOODS

Chunky Monkey F-Factor Smoothie

Pumpkin Spice Overnight Oats

Breakfast Burritos

Banana Chocolate Chip Muffins

Italian Herb Frittata

The F-Factor Breakfast Sandwich

### SOUPS, SALADS, AND VEGETABLES

Moroccan Lentil Soup

Black Bean Soup

Minestrone Soup

Tanya's House Salad

Asian Chicken Salad

Lettuce-less Greek Salad

Roasted Corn Salsa

Cauliflower "Fried Rice"

Sweet Potato Chips

Spiced Garbanzo Beans

### CHICKEN AND TURKEY MAIN DISHES

Scallion and Ginger Spiced Chicken

Crispy Pecan Chicken

Chicken Ratatouille

Roasted Chicken Harvest Bowl

Turkey Chili

### BEEF, PORK, AND LAMB MAIN DISHES

Easy Beef Fajitas

Wholesome Sloppy Joes

Grilled Beef and Bean Burgers

Best Meat Loaf

Zucchini Noodle Bolognese

### FISH AND SHELLFISH MAIN DISHES

Crispy Oven-Fried Fish

Tuna and White Bean Salad

Broiled Snapper with Black Bean Salsa

Zesty Shrimp Burritos

Thai Shrimp Summer Rolls

### PASTA AND GRAINS

Pasta Bolognese

Macaroni and Cheese

Linguine with Clam Sauce

Nutty Stir-Fried Rice

Quinoa and Chickpea Burgers in Lettuce
　　Wraps

Tabouli Salad

### SWEETS

Chocolate-Cherry-Almond Biscotti

Cinnamon Sugar Skinny Chips

Cranberry-Walnut Chutney

Berry Crisp

Chocolate-Covered Bananas

✳ BREAKFAST FOODS

# Berry Breakfast Parfait

STEPS 1, 2, AND 3

*When made in a large stemmed glass, this looks pretty enough to serve to guests.*

> 1 container (5.3 oz) 0% fat Greek or Icelandic yogurt
> ½ cup strawberries, sliced
> ⅓ cup All-Bran Bran Buds
> ¼ cup blueberries
> 1 tablespoon sliced almonds
> cinnamon (optional)

1. In a dish or tall glass, spoon ⅓ of the yogurt.
2. Top with strawberries and then half of the All-Bran Bran Buds.
3. Repeat layer, but use blueberries for the fruit. Top off with last ⅓ of yogurt.
4. Top with sliced almonds and sprinkle with cinnamon if desired.

SERVES 1

**THE F-FACTOR DIET NUTRITIONAL CONTENT FOR JOURNALING**
Per Serving: 37 g carbohydrate • 16 g fiber

**ACTUAL NUTRITIONAL CONTENT**
Per Serving: 246 calories • 42 g carbohydrate • 16 g fiber • 20 g protein • 5 g total fat •
0 g sat. fat • 261 mg sodium

RECIPES

# Strawberry F-Factor Smoothie

STEPS 1, 2, AND 3

*Strawberries and cream! This delicious smoothie fills you up for few calories. It's fruity, refreshing, and a great way to start your day.*

> 1 cup crushed ice
> 1¼ cup frozen strawberries
> ½ cup unsweetened almond milk
> 1–2 scoops F-Factor Vanilla Fiber/Protein Powder
> Truvia

1. Place all the ingredients in a blender. Mix on high speed until well blended.
2. Pour into a glass and serve.

SERVES 1

**THE F-FACTOR DIET NUTRITIONAL CONTENT FOR JOURNALING**
Per Serving: 40 g carbohydrate • 24 g fiber

**ACTUAL NUTRITIONAL CONTENT**
Per Serving: 205 calories • 41 g carbohydrate • 24 g fiber • 21 g protein • 3 g total fat • 0 g sat. fat • 78 mg sodium

# F-Factor's Famous High-Fiber Pancakes

STEPS 1, 2, AND 3

*One short-stack coming right up! Serve with Walden Farms "Calorie Free" Pancake Syrup for a real high-fiber treat that's 100% #FFACTORAPPROVED.*

> 4 GG Bran Crispbreads, pulverized into sprinkles
> Egg whites of 4 large eggs
> 1 teaspoon vanilla extract
> ¼ teaspoon cinnamon
> 1–2 packets Truvia, as needed
> nonstick cooking spray

1. In a blender pulverize GGs into GG sprinkles.
2. Add egg whites, vanilla, cinnamon, and sweetener (if using) to blender and pulse until ingredients are well combined into a batter.
3. Spray pan with nonstick cooking spray and place over medium heat.
4. Pour mix into pan to create 1–3 pancakes of desired size and cook until edges begin to brown. Flip and cook for another few minutes.
5. Top with syrup or fresh fruit, as desired, and enjoy.

SERVES 1

**THE F-FACTOR DIET NUTRITIONAL CONTENT FOR JOURNALING**
Per Serving: 24 g carbohydrate • 16 g fiber

**ACTUAL NUTRITIONAL CONTENT**
Per Serving: 165 calories • 24 g carbohydrate • 16 g fiber • 19 g protein • 0g fat • 0 g sat. fat • 1 mg sodium

## Greek Omelet

STEPS 1, 2, AND 3

*This is one of my favorite breakfasts. The saltiness of the cheese balances the sweetness of the vegetables. Eat with 4 high-fiber crackers on Step 1 or add a piece of whole-wheat toast on Step 2.*

nonstick cooking spray
¼ cup diced onions
8 mushrooms, sliced
1 cup spinach, raw
1 plum tomato, cubed
1 egg and 2 egg whites, beaten with a dash of salt and pepper
1 ounce feta cheese, crumbled

1. Heat a nonstick pan and spray with nonstick cooking spray.
2. Add onions, and sauté until translucent, approximately 3 minutes.
3. Add mushrooms, and cook for 2 minutes more.
4. Add spinach and tomato and cook until spinach is wilted.

5. Pour eggs over vegetables and tilt pan until the eggs cover the entire surface.

6. Sprinkle cheese over top and when eggs are set, fold omelet in half and serve.

SERVES 1

**THE F-FACTOR DIET NUTRITIONAL CONTENT FOR JOURNALING**
Per Serving: 0 g carbohydrate • 4 g fiber

**ACTUAL NUTRITIONAL CONTENT**
Per Serving: 253 calories • 16 g carbohydrate • 4 g fiber • 23 g protein • 12 g total fat •
6 g sat. fat • 525 mg sodium

# Apple Cinnamon "Oatmeal"

STEPS 1, 2, AND 3

*Jazz up your boring bowl of oats with this fiber-filled alternative. Not an apple fan? Raspberries, blueberries, peaches, or pears work well, too!*

1 cup apple, diced (½ medium apple)
dash of cinnamon
⅓ cup All-Bran Bran Buds or ½ cup Nature's Path SmartBran
  cereal
⅓ cup unsweetened almond milk
⅓ cup water

1. Place a saucepan over medium-high heat. Add 1–2 tablespoons water and diced apples. Add dash of cinnamon and cook for 2 minutes, while stirring.

2. When apples have softened, add cereal, almond milk, and water. Stir and cook for 3 minutes, continually stirring.

3. Add another 2 tablespoons of water and cook until all the water has been absorbed and the consistency mimics oatmeal.

4. Spoon mixture into bowl and serve immediately.

SERVES 1

**THE F-FACTOR DIET NUTRITIONAL CONTENT FOR JOURNALING**
Per Serving: 35 g carbohydrate • 15 g fiber

**ACTUAL NUTRITIONAL CONTENT**
Per Serving: 140 calories • 36 g carbohydrate • 15 g fiber • 3 g protein • 2 g fat • 0 g sat. fat •
202 mg sodium

# Heart Healthy Turkey Sausage

STEPS 1, 2, AND 3

*After making your own sausage, you may never go back to store-bought. These
are simple and delicious and contain half the fat of regular sausage!*

  1 pound ground turkey
  2 teaspoons paprika
  1 teaspoon ground sage
  1 teaspoon dried thyme
  ¼ teaspoon ground fresh nutmeg
  ½ teaspoon ground black pepper
  1 teaspoon Kosher salt
  nonstick cooking spray

1. Combine all ingredients in a large bowl, using your hands to gently blend
   the mixture.
2. Divide the sausage mixture into 12 pieces and form into patties.
3. Heat a heavy nonstick skillet and spray with nonstick cooking spray.
4. Cook the sausage through, about 5 minutes on each side.

MAKES 12 PATTIES; SERVES 4

**THE F-FACTOR DIET NUTRITIONAL CONTENT FOR JOURNALING**
Per Serving: 0 g carbohydrate • 0 g fiber

**ACTUAL NUTRITIONAL CONTENT**
Per Serving: 57 calories • 0 g carbohydrate • 0 g fiber • 7 g protein • 3 g total fat • 1 g
sat. fat • 229 mg sodium

RECIPES

# Chicken Soup

STEPS 1, 2, AND 3

*Many soup recipes call for homemade stock. Stock adds undeniable flavor, but it can also take hours to prepare. Instead, I rely on canned chicken broth for ease and convenience. The dill gives this soup a special flavor.*

1 small onion, diced

2 cloves garlic, minced

4 carrots, peeled and diced

2 parsnips, peeled and diced

4 stalks celery, chopped

1 pound skinless chicken cutlets, diced into bite-sized pieces

1 tablespoon fresh dill, chopped

½ teaspoon salt

½ teaspoon pepper

4 cups chicken broth

2 cups water

nonstick cooking spray

1. Heat a large stockpot over high heat. Spray with cooking spray.
2. Add the onion and sauté for 2 minutes. Add the garlic and sauté for 2 minutes more.
3. Add the carrots, parsnips, celery, chicken, dill, salt, pepper, broth, and water.
4. Bring the mixture to a boil and then reduce heat to a simmer for 20 minutes. Serve.

SERVES 8

**THE F-FACTOR DIET NUTRITIONAL CONTENT FOR JOURNALING**
Per Serving: 0 g carbohydrate • 2 g fiber

**ACTUAL NUTRITIONAL CONTENT**
Per Serving: 114 calories • 8 g carbohydrate • 2 g fiber • 16 g protein • 2 g total fat • 0 g sat. fat • 592 mg sodium

RECIPES

# Vegetable Soup

*The many vegetables in this soup make it incredibly filling. Feel free to add your favorite vegetables or leave out ones you don't like.*

1 onion, diced

2 cloves garlic, minced

2 cups peeled baby carrots, cut into bite-sized pieces

1 head of celery hearts, cut into bite-sized pieces

1 box button mushrooms, sliced

2 zucchini, diced into bite-sized pieces

1 16-ounce can crushed tomatoes

4 cups chicken broth

1 teaspoon dried basil

1 teaspoon dried oregano

salt and pepper

2 cups frozen broccoli florets

2 cups frozen spinach

Parmesan cheese

nonstick cooking spray

1. Heat a large stockpot over high heat. Spray with cooking spray.
2. Add the onion and sauté for 2 minutes. Add the garlic and sauté for 2 minutes more.
3. Add the carrots, celery, mushrooms, zucchini, tomatoes, chicken broth, and herbs. Season with salt and pepper.
4. Bring the mixture to a boil and then simmer for 15 minutes.
5. Add the broccoli and spinach and cook for 5 more minutes.
6. Serve and top with grated Parmesan cheese.

SERVES 8

**THE F-FACTOR DIET NUTRITIONAL CONTENT FOR JOURNALING**
Per Serving: 0 g carbohydrate • 7 g fiber

RECIPES

**ACTUAL NUTRITIONAL CONTENT**
Per Serving: 124 calories • 21 g carbohydrate • 7 g fiber • 8 g protein • 2 g total fat • 1 g sat.
fat • 602 mg sodium

# Cabbage Soup

STEPS 1, 2, AND 3

*Who can forget the cabbage soup diet? While this recipe is tastier than the original,
one thing remains the same—it is still low in calories!*

6 carrots, peeled and diced
6 scallions, chopped
1 16-ounce can crushed tomatoes
1 large head green cabbage, chopped fine
2 cups fresh green beans, ends removed, chopped into bite-sized pieces
1 bunch celery, cut into bite-sized pieces
2 cups mushrooms, sliced
1 32-ounce box chicken broth
salt and pepper

1. Place all the vegetables in a large pot. Add the chicken broth and enough
   water to cover. Season with salt and pepper.
2. Bring the mixture to a boil over high heat and cook for 10 minutes. Reduce
   heat and simmer until the vegetables are tender.

SERVES 8

**THE F-FACTOR DIET NUTRITIONAL CONTENT FOR JOURNALING**
Per Serving: 0 g carbohydrate • 9 g fiber

**ACTUAL NUTRITIONAL CONTENT**
Per Serving: 128 calories • 25 g carbohydrate • 9 g fiber • 8 g protein • 1 g total fat • 0 g sat.
fat • 505 mg sodium

# Grilled Sirloin Salad

STEPS 1, 2, AND 3

*Why have a plain bowl of salad when you can feast on grilled spiced sirloin and greens? This salad is hearty enough to serve for dinner.*

1 clove garlic, chopped
2 tablespoons reduced-sodium soy sauce
2 tablespoons balsamic vinegar
2 tablespoons peanut oil
1 tablespoon Truvia
1 teaspoon chopped fresh ginger
¾ pound sirloin, trimmed of fat
salt and pepper to taste
8 scallions
12 cups mesclun greens
1 red bell pepper, seeded and sliced into thin strips

1. Heat a grill pan.
2. In a blender or food processor, combine garlic, soy sauce, vinegar, oil, Truvia, and ginger; blend until smooth. Set aside.
3. Season beef with salt and pepper.
4. Grill sirloin and scallions until meat is medium rare and scallions are slightly charred, about 6 to 8 minutes.
5. Let sirloin rest for 5 minutes before slicing. Cut against the grain into very thin slices. Cut scallions into 1-inch pieces.
6. In a large bowl, toss greens and red bell pepper strips with reserved dressing. Arrange on a platter and top with sirloin and grilled scallions.
7. Serve immediately.

SERVES 4

**THE F-FACTOR DIET NUTRITIONAL CONTENT FOR JOURNALING**
Per Serving: 0 g carbohydrate • 2 g fiber

RECIPES

**ACTUAL NUTRITIONAL CONTENT**
Per Serving: 196 calories • 6 g carbohydrate • 2 g fiber • 21 g protein • 10 g total fat • 2 g
sat. fat • 453 mg sodium

# Tuna-Egg Salad

STEPS 1, 2, AND 3

*The addition of egg whites adds volume and extra protein, without adding fat
or excess calories. Try this salad on top of high-fiber crackers for a delicious afternoon snack, or place a scoop on top of a salad for a satisfying lunch.*

    1 12-ounce can tuna fish, canned in water
    6 eggs
    2 celery stalks
    ½ cup diced Vidalia onion
    3 tablespoons low-fat mayonnaise
    salt and pepper

1. Drain tuna fish and break up with a fork.
2. Place eggs in a pot of boiling water and cook for 10 minutes, until hard-boiled.
3. While the eggs are cooking, finely dice the celery and onion; add to tuna.
4. When the eggs are ready, rinse under cold water, and remove the shells. Discard the egg yolks and finely chop the egg whites. Add to tuna mixture.
5. Add mayonnaise and mix well. Add salt and pepper to taste.
6. Serve.

SERVES 4

**THE F-FACTOR DIET NUTRITIONAL CONTENT FOR JOURNALING**
Per Serving: 0 g carbohydrate • 1 g fiber

**ACTUAL NUTRITIONAL CONTENT**
Per Serving: 128 calories • 3 g carbohydrate • 1 g fiber • 25 g protein • 1 g total fat • 0 g
sat. fat • 570 mg sodium

# Spinach Salad with Warm Bacon Vinaigrette

STEPS 1, 2, AND 3

*This salad is a lighter version of an old favorite. Friends rave when I serve it. To turn it into a meal, add grilled chicken or shrimp on top.*

3 strips of turkey bacon
2 tablespoons olive oil
2 tablespoons red wine vinegar
1 teaspoon Dijon mustard
1 garlic clove, minced
salt and pepper
1 bag baby spinach, prewashed
1 small pear,
    cut into bite-sized pieces
1 ounce Romano cheese,
    shaved into thin slices

1. Cook the bacon in a skillet over medium heat until crisp and brown, 6 to 8 minutes. Drain on a paper towel and break into small pieces. Set aside.
2. Add olive oil to the pan and whisk in the vinegar, mustard, minced garlic, and a dash of salt and pepper. Add the bacon and set aside.
3. In a large bowl, combine the spinach and pear. Spoon the warm bacon vinaigrette over the spinach and toss to coat. Add cheese and serve.

SERVES 4

**THE F-FACTOR DIET NUTRITIONAL CONTENT FOR JOURNALING**
Per Serving: 4 g carbohydrate • 3 g fiber

**ACTUAL NUTRITIONAL CONTENT**
Per Serving: 157 calories • 9 g carbohydrate • 3 g fiber • 7 g protein • 11 g total fat • 3 g sat. fat • 411 mg sodium

RECIPES

# String Beans in Tomato Sauce

*A version of this dish can be found at some of my favorite restaurants . . .
Amaranth, Freds at Barneys New York, and Avra Madison. If you are not in
New York City, don't sweat it—now you, too, can enjoy this dish.*

1 pound string beans, washed, with ends trimmed
1 teaspoon olive oil
4 cloves garlic, sliced
1 large shallot, diced
1 cup cherry tomatoes, sliced
2 tablespoons tomato paste
½ cup Rao's Marinara or Tomato Basil Sauce
salt and pepper, to taste
1 tablespoon red pepper flakes

1. Wash and trim ends of string beans. Cut in half and place aside.
2. in a large pan over medium heat, add 1 teaspoon olive oil, garlic, and diced shallots, and sauté until translucent.
3. Add the sliced cherry tomatoes and cook until juices are released.
4. Add 2 tablespoons tomato paste and sauté for another 2 to 4 minutes, stirring occasionally.
5. Stir in tomato sauce. Add string beans, stir, and cover for 20 minutes or until string beans are tender.
6. Remove from heat, season with salt and pepper to taste.
7. Transfer to a platter and sprinkle red pepper flakes. Serve immediately.

SERVES 4

**THE F-FACTOR DIET NUTRITIONAL CONTENT FOR JOURNALING**
Per Serving: 3 g carbohydrate • 5 g fiber

**ACTUAL NUTRITIONAL CONTENT**
Per Serving: 75 calories • 15 g carbohydrate • 5 g fiber • 3 g protein • 1 g fat • 0 g sat. fat • 160 mg sodium

# Broccoli Sesame Salad

*This salad goes well with grilled fish. You can substitute frozen broccoli if fresh isn't available.*

    4 cups broccoli florets
    2 teaspoons canola oil
    1 tablespoon rice wine vinegar
    1½ teaspoons low-sodium soy sauce
    ¼ cup chopped scallions
    2 teaspoons toasted sesame seeds

1. Place broccoli in a small microwave container and fill with ½ inch water. Cook on full power for 3 minutes until crisp and tender.
2. Rinse immediately with cool running water and drain well in a colander.
3. Place broccoli in a bowl and add the rest of the ingredients. Stir well and serve immediately or chill for later use.

SERVES 4

**THE F-FACTOR DIET NUTRITIONAL CONTENT FOR JOURNALING**
Per serving: 0 g carbohydrate • 3 g fiber

**ACTUAL NUTRITIONAL CONTENT**
Per Serving: 55 calories • 5 g carbohydrate • 3 g fiber • 3 g protein • 3 g total fat • 0 g sat. fat • 260 mg sodium

# Eggplant Rollatini

*Eggplant rollatini is a decadent Italian dish and one of my favorites—best part about my version is that, unlike the traditional one, it's completely guilt-free. Mangia!*

2 medium Italian eggplants, cut lengthwise into 10 (¼-inch-thick)
    slices (21 ounces total when sliced)
kosher salt and fresh black pepper, to taste
1½ cups Rao's Marinara Sauce
1 large egg
½ cup part skim ricotta cheese
½ cup grated Pecorino Romano cheese
1 8-ounce package frozen spinach, heated through and squeezed well
1 clove garlic, minced
1 cup shredded part-skim mozzarella

1. Cut the 2 ends off the eggplants. Cut the eggplants lengthwise, into
   ¼-inch-thick slices, until you have a total of 10 slices about the same size.
   It's easiest to do this with a mandoline.
2. Sprinkle the eggplant with kosher salt to help remove excess moisture and
   bitterness from the eggplant. Set aside for about 10 to 15 minutes. Pat dry
   with a towel.
3. Preheat oven to 400°F. Season the eggplant with a little more salt and
   pepper, then arrange on two parchment-lined baking sheets. Cover tightly
   with foil and bake until eggplant is tender but not fully cooked, about 8
   to 10 minutes.
4. Spread ¼ cup marinara sauce on the bottom of a 13-by-9-inch baking
   dish.
5. In a medium bowl, beat the egg, then mix together with ricotta, Pecorino
   Romano, spinach, garlic, ¼ teaspoon salt and ⅛ teaspoon pepper.
6. Pat eggplant dry with paper towels. Spoon 2 generous tablespoons of the
   ricotta-spinach mixture onto one end of each eggplant slice, spreading to
   cover. Starting at the short end, roll up slices and arrange them each seam-
   side down in the prepared dish. Top with remaining marinara sauce and
   mozzarella cheese and tightly cover with foil.
7. Bake until the eggplant is very tender, about 1 hour.
8. Remove from oven and let cool 5 minutes before serving.

**THE F-FACTOR DIET NUTRITIONAL CONTENT FOR JOURNALING**
Per Serving: 3 g carbohydrate • 5 g fiber

**ACTUAL NUTRITIONAL CONTENT**
Per Serving: 169 calories • 13 g carbohydrate • 5 g fiber • 13 g protein • 8 g fat • 4 g sat.
fat • 327 mg sodium

# Blackened Green Beans

STEP 1, 2, AND 3

*For years, blackened broccoli was all the rage. but wait until you try my black-
ened green beans. Take a seat, broccoli, it's green beans' turn to shine . . . or
blacken.*

> **1 10.8-ounce bag frozen premium whole green beans**
> **2 cloves garlic, minced**
> **1 tablespoon olive oil**
> **salt to taste**

1. Add a bag of frozen green beans and minced garlic to a pan and place over
   medium-low heat.
2. Drizzle with 1 tablespoon olive oil, mixing to coat beans and garlic. Sprinkle with salt.
3. Cover and cook for 15 minutes.
4. Uncover and cook for an additional 30 to 45 minutes, stirring occasionally.
5. When green beans have achieved desired level of char, remove from heat
   and serve.

SERVES 2

**THE F-FACTOR DIET NUTRITIONAL CONTENT FOR JOURNALING**
Per Serving: 0 g carbohydrate • 5 g fiber

**ACTUAL NUTRITIONAL CONTENT**
Per Serving: 113 calories • 12 g carbohydrate • 5 g fiber • 3 g protein • 7 g fat • 1 g sat.
fat • 242 mg sodium

# Roasted Brussels Sprouts

STEPS 1, 2, AND 3

*Roasting Brussels sprouts brings out their natural sweetness. For those who don't like Brussels sprouts, I say give this recipe a try. You might become a convert!*

> 2 cups chicken broth
> 1 10-ounce package frozen no-salt-added Brussels sprouts, thawed
> 1 tablespoon olive oil
> 1 tablespoon chopped garlic
> ½ teaspoon salt
> ¼ teaspoon pepper
> 2 tablespoons sliced almonds, toasted

1. Preheat oven to broil.
2. Place chicken broth in a pot and bring to a boil. Add Brussels sprouts and cook for 5 minutes, until tender.
3. Drain Brussels sprouts. Cut Brussels sprouts in half and place in a bowl. Add chopped oil, garlic, salt, and pepper and toss evenly to coat.
4. Spread Brussels sprouts onto a baking sheet and broil for 8 minutes, stirring after 4 minutes to ensure even cooking. Brussels sprouts should be browned on the edges.
5. Top with sliced almonds and serve.

SERVES 4

**THE F-FACTOR DIET NUTRITIONAL CONTENT FOR JOURNALING**
Per Serving: 0 g carbohydrate • 3 g fiber

**ACTUAL NUTRITIONAL CONTENT**
Per Serving: 99 calories • 8 g carbohydrate • 3 g fiber • 6 g protein • 6 g total fat • 1 g sat. fat • 686 mg sodium

# Cauliflower Pizza Crust

*First step to a high-protein, low-carb, cauliflower pizza is a good cauliflower pizza crust. Prepare and top as you wish!*

> 1 large-sized cauliflower head (should yield 2–3 cups once riced/processed)
> ¼ teaspoon kosher salt
> ½ teaspoon dried basil
> ½ teaspoon dried oregano
> ½ teaspoon garlic powder
> ¼ cup grated Parmesan cheese
> 1 cup shredded part-skim mozzarella cheese
> 1 egg
> nonstick cooking oil

1. Preheat oven to 450°F. If using a pizza stone, place it in the oven to heat.
2. Place a large piece of parchment paper on a cutting board and spray it with nonstick cooking oil. If not using a pizza stone, line a baking sheet with oiled parchment paper and set aside.
3. Place the riced cauliflower "snow" in a microwave-safe bowl, cover with plastic wrap, and microwave for 2 to 3 minutes.
4. Dump cooked cauliflower onto a clean tea towel and allow to cool for a few minutes. Once cauliflower is cool enough to handle, either wrap it up in the dish towel and wring it to squeeze the water out, or place in a colander and push down on it with a towel. It is important to get as much water out as possible to ensure your crust comes out crispy, instead of a crumbly mess.
5. In a large bowl, mix up your strained cauliflower rice with the remaining ingredients. Mix well until a "dough" is formed.
6. Press the dough out into a crust on your oiled parchment paper. Pat it down into a thin circle. If using a baking sheet, place in oven.
7. If using a pizza stone, slide the parchment paper onto the heated stone in the oven.

RECIPES

8. Bake for 8 to 11 minutes. The crust should be firm and golden brown when finished. Remove from oven.
9. Top pizza as desired, place back in oven for an additional 5 to 7 minutes (until toppings are cooked to desired doneness), slice and serve.

SERVES 4

**THE F-FACTOR DIET NUTRITIONAL CONTENT FOR JOURNALING**
Per Serving: 3 g carbohydrate • 4 g fiber

**ACTUAL NUTRITIONAL CONTENT**
Per Serving: 147 calories • 11 g carbohydrate • 4 g fiber • 11 g protein • 7 g fat • 3 g sat. fat • 423 mg sodium

## Sautéed Zucchini with Parmesan

STEPS 1, 2, AND 3

*Who knew something so cheesy could be good for you?*

2 teaspoons extra-virgin olive oil
2 pounds zucchini (about 4 medium), sliced ¼ inch thick
⅛ teaspoon salt
freshly ground pepper to taste
½ cup finely shredded Parmesan cheese

1. Preheat broiler.
2. Heat oil in a large nonstick skillet over medium heat.
3. Add zucchini and cook, stirring every 2 to 3 minutes, until tender and most of the slices are golden brown. Season with salt and pepper.
4. Spread zucchini in an even layer in ovensafe pie plate. Sprinkle with Parmesan and broil for 2 to 3 minutes, until cheese melts and bubbles.
5. Cut into wedges and serve.

**THE F-FACTOR DIET NUTRITIONAL CONTENT FOR JOURNALING**
Per Serving: 0 g carbohydrate • 2 g fiber

**ACTUAL NUTRITIONAL CONTENT**
Per Serving: 113 calories • 5 g carbohydrate • 2 g fiber • 9 g protein • 7 g total fat • 4 g sat.
fat • 403 mg sodium

# Four Pepper Sauté

STEPS 1, 2, AND 3

*This dish is colorful, sweet, crunchy, and amazingly low in calories.*

> 1 teaspoon extra-virgin olive oil
> 1 yellow pepper, seeded and cut into thin strips
> 1 red pepper, seeded and cut into thin strips
> 1 orange pepper, seeded and cut into thin strips
> 1 green pepper, seeded and cut into thin strips
> 1 red onion, peeled and thinly sliced
> 2 garlic cloves, finely chopped
> 1 tablespoon Worcestershire sauce
> 1 tablespoon water
> ¼ teaspoon freshly ground pepper

1. Heat oil in a nonstick 10-inch skillet. Add peppers, onion, and garlic and sauté for 5 minutes.
2. Add the Worcestershire sauce and water, and cook over medium heat for 2 minutes, stirring frequently.
3. Add the ground pepper, stir, and serve.

SERVES 4

**THE F-FACTOR DIET NUTRITIONAL CONTENT FOR JOURNALING**
Per Serving: 0 g carbohydrate • 3 g fiber

RECIPES

**ACTUAL NUTRITIONAL CONTENT**
Per Serving: 75 calories • 13 g carbohydrate • 3 g fiber • 2 g protein • 2 g total fat • 0 g sat.
fat • 63 mg sodium

RECIPES

✳ CHICKEN AND TURKEY MAIN DISHES

# Tandoori Chicken

STEPS 1, 2, AND 3

*If you're a serious lover of Indian food, you will adore this dish!*

3 garlic cloves, chopped
1 teaspoon ground cumin
½ teaspoon cayenne pepper
1 teaspoon turmeric
1 tablespoon chopped fresh ginger
1 tablespoon fresh lime juice
½ teaspoon salt
8 ounces 0% fat Greek yogurt
4 4-ounce boneless, skinless chicken breasts

1. In a large bowl, combine all ingredients except chicken and mix well.
2. Add chicken and marinate in the refrigerator for 24 hours. Remove the chicken and discard the marinade.
3. Preheat the broiler or a grill pan on the stovetop.
4. Broil or grill the chicken 5 minutes per side.

SERVES 4

**THE F-FACTOR DIET NUTRITIONAL CONTENT FOR JOURNALING**
Per Serving: 0 g carbohydrate • 0 g fiber

**ACTUAL NUTRITIONAL CONTENT**
Per Serving: 220 calories • 3 g carbohydrate • 0 g fiber • 40 g protein • 4 g total fat • 1 g sat.
fat • 636 mg sodium

# Poached Chicken Salad with Raspberry Vinaigrette

STEPS 1, 2, AND 3

*This salad makes a wonderful weekend lunch or a light summer supper.*

- 4 cups canned chicken stock (preferably nonfat)
- 1 pound boneless, skinless chicken breasts
- 1 14-ounce can artichoke hearts, drained
- 1 tablespoon olive oil
- 2 tablespoons raspberry vinegar
- 1 tablespoon water
- ½ pint fresh raspberries
- 8 cups mesclun greens

1. In a medium sauté pan, bring chicken stock to a simmer and add chicken breasts. Poach the chicken for about 6 minutes, turning to cook through. Remove chicken from pan with a slotted spoon and set aside to cool.
2. Slice the artichoke hearts into bite-sized pieces.
3. Cut the cooled chicken into strips.
4. In a blender, combine olive oil, vinegar, water, and ½ cup raspberries, and purée until smooth.
5. Divide mesclun greens, chicken, artichokes, remaining raspberries, and dressing among 4 plates.

SERVES 4

**THE F-FACTOR DIET NUTRITIONAL CONTENT FOR JOURNALING**
Per Serving: 4 g carbohydrate • 5 g fiber

**ACTUAL NUTRITIONAL CONTENT**
Per Serving: 315 calories • 14 g carbohydrate • 5 g fiber • 43 g protein • 9 g total fat • 2 g sat. fat • 1170 mg sodium

RECIPES

# Turkey Meat Loaf

*This modern take on traditional turkey meat loaf is so easy to make and always a crowd-pleaser.*

1 1-pound package lean (97%) ground turkey breast

2 eggs

½ cup artichoke salsa (you can use regular salsa if you can't find artichoke salsa)

¼ cup red bell pepper, chopped

¼ cup yellow bell pepper, chopped

½ cup onion, chopped

3 GG Bran Crispbreads, pulverized into sprinkles

1 teaspoon garlic powder

salt and pepper to taste

1.  Preheat oven to 350° F.
2.  In a large bowl combine the turkey, eggs, salsa, red bell pepper, yellow bell pepper, onion, GG sprinkles, garlic powder, and salt and pepper to taste. Mix well with hands until blended.
3.  Roll into a small loaf and place on a foil-lined baking sheet.
4.  Bake in the preheated oven for 25 minutes.

SERVES 4

**THE F-FACTOR DIET NUTRITIONAL CONTENT FOR JOURNALING**
Per Serving: 5 g carbohydrate • 4 g fiber

**ACTUAL NUTRITIONAL CONTENT**
Per Serving: 242 calories • 9 g carbohydrate • 4 g fiber • 26 g protein • 12 g fat • 3 g sat. fat • 249 mg sodium

# Guiltless Chicken Parmesan

*Oh, how my family loves chicken parm, but the classic version has almost 30 grams of carbs per serving and no fiber. My version is fiber-packed and pleases even the pickiest eaters.*

nonstick cooking spray
6 GG Bran Crispbreads, pulverized into sprinkles
1 tablespoon Italian seasoning
1 teaspoon garlic powder
½ teaspoon salt
¼ teaspoon pepper
½ cup (8 tablespoons) grated Parmesan cheese
½ cup Egg Beaters
4 4-ounce boneless skinless chicken breasts (raw)
1 cup Rao's Marinara Sauce

1. Preheat oven to 400° F. Spray a large baking sheet with nonstick cooking spray.
2. Combine GG sprinkles, Italian seasoning, garlic powder, salt, and pepper with ½ the Parmesan cheese in a bowl. Set aside. Pour Egg Beaters into a separate bowl and place beside dry-mixture bowl.
3. One at a time, dip each chicken breast into Egg Beaters, and then into the dry mixture to coat both sides, before placing on baking sheet.
4. Repeat step 3 with remaining chicken breasts.
5. Spoon half the marinara sauce atop each chicken breast and place baking sheet in oven.
6. Bake for 15 minutes, remove from oven, and flip each breast over. Spoon remaining tomato sauce over the top of each breast. Sprinkle remaining Parmesan cheese atop them and place baking sheet back in oven to bake for another 15 minutes, or until cheese is melted.

RECIPES

SERVES 4

**THE F-FACTOR DIET NUTRITIONAL CONTENT FOR JOURNALING**
Per Serving: 14 g carbohydrate • 7 g fiber

**ACTUAL NUTRITIONAL CONTENT**
Per Serving: 302 calories • 17 g carbohydrate • 7 g fiber • 24 g protein • 8 g fat • 4 g sat.
fat • 597 mg sodium

# Southwest Turkey Burgers

STEPS 1, 2, AND 3

*Lean ground turkey meat can taste bland. All the bold herbs and spices kick up
the flavor in these burgers.*

> 1 pound lean ground turkey
> 2 cloves garlic, finely chopped
> 2 tablespoons chopped cilantro
> ½ red pepper, finely chopped
> 1 jalapeño pepper finely chopped (optional)
> 2 teaspoons ground cumin
> 1 teaspoon chili powder
> 1 teaspoon salt

1. Combine all the ingredients and divide mixture into four patties.
2. Heat a grill or a grill pan and cook burgers to desired doneness (approximately 3 minutes per side for medium).

SERVES 4

**THE F-FACTOR DIET NUTRITIONAL CONTENT FOR JOURNALING**
Per Serving: 1 g carbohydrate • 0 g fiber

**ACTUAL NUTRITIONAL CONTENT**
Per Serving: 183 calories • 1 g carbohydrate • 0 g fiber • 34 g protein • 4 g total fat • 1 g
sat. fat • 626 mg sodium

# Classic Steak House Filet Mignon

STEPS 1, 2, AND 3

*There's nothing more delicious than a perfectly cooked steak. And since filet mignon is a lean cut, you get to enjoy the flavor without all the fat and calories of fattier cuts.*

2 teaspoons black peppercorns
¼ teaspoon dried rosemary
1 teaspoon dry mustard
1 teaspoon Kosher salt
½ teaspoon garlic powder
4 4-ounce beef tenderloin steaks, trimmed
cooking oil spray

1. Prepare grill.
2. Place peppercorns and rosemary in a spice grinder and pulse (or use a mortar and pestle to grind).
3. Combine pepper mixture, mustard powder, salt, and garlic powder and rub evenly over both sides of the steaks.
4. Place steaks on a grill rack coated with cooking spray and grill for 3 minutes on each side (for medium rare). Cook longer if you desire the meat more well done.

SERVES 4

**THE F-FACTOR DIET NUTRITIONAL CONTENT FOR JOURNALING**
Per Serving: 0 g carbohydrates • 0 g fiber

**ACTUAL NUTRITIONAL CONTENT**
Per Serving: 175 calories • 0 g carbohydrate • 0 g fiber • 24 g protein • 8 g total fat • 3 g sat. fat • 643 mg sodium

RECIPES

# TZ's Mozzarella-Stuffed Meatballs

*Can you say ooey-gooey deliciousness? The flavorful surprise of cheese oozing out of every tasty bite makes this an instant crowd-pleaser.*

**2 pounds 97% lean beef**
**10 GG Bran Crispbreads, pulverized into sprinkles**
**½ cup grated Parmesan cheese**
**½ cup water**
**1 large Vidalia onion, minced**
**1 clove garlic, minced**
**1 teaspoon onion powder**
**1 teaspoon kosher salt**
**1 tablespoon Italian seasoning**
**1 large egg, lightly beaten**
**8 part-skim mozzarella string cheese sticks, cut into fifths (40 pieces total)**

1. Preheat oven to 400°F. Line 2 baking sheets with parchment paper or tinfoil and set aside.
2. In a large bowl, combine all ingredients except mozzarella cheese; mix well.
3. Using a scoop, divide mixture into 40 meatballs and place on a baking sheet or plate. One at a time, place each meatball in the palm of your cupped hand. Press mozzarella cube into meatball and roll back into a ball, making sure to cover cheese completely.
4. Place on prepared baking sheets. Bake for 35 minutes, rotating trays halfway through cook time.
5. Serve immediately.

SERVES 10 (4 MEATBALLS EACH)

**THE F-FACTOR DIET NUTRITIONAL CONTENT FOR JOURNALING**
Per Serving: 8 g carbohydrate • 4 g fiber

# Greek-Style Pork

*This stew will impart a delicious aroma in your home. Serve it with whole-wheat pita on step 2.*

    1 pound boneless pork tenderloin
    ½ medium onion, cut into wedges
    ½ green bell pepper, diced
    1 14½-ounce can diced tomatoes
    ½ teaspoon dried oregano
    ½ teaspoon salt
    ¼ teaspoon pepper
    ½ teaspoon ground cinnamon
    2 ounces feta cheese
    cooking spray

1. Trim any fat from the pork. Cut into ½-inch cubes.
2. In a large nonstick skillet sprayed with cooking spray, brown the pork, onion, and pepper. Drain off any fat.
3. Stir in undrained tomatoes, oregano, salt, pepper, and cinnamon. Bring to a boil. Reduce heat, cover, and simmer for 25 minutes.
4. Sprinkle feta cheese over pork and serve immediately.

SERVES 4

**THE F-FACTOR DIET NUTRITIONAL CONTENT FOR JOURNALING**
Per Serving: 0 g carbohydrate • 2 g fiber

**ACTUAL NUTRITIONAL CONTENT**
Per Serving: 227 calories • 7 g carbohydrate • 2 g fiber • 28 g protein • 9 g total fat • 4 g
sat. fat • 510 mg sodium

# Broiled Baby Lamb Chops

*Baby lamb chops are my father's all-time favorite food. This one is for you, Dad!*

1 tablespoon fresh rosemary, chopped
3 cloves garlic, minced
1 tablespoon fresh lemon juice
2 tablespoons olive oil
8 baby rib lamb chops (about 1½ to 2 pounds)
salt and pepper

1. Mix the rosemary, garlic, lemon juice, and olive oil in a large plastic Ziploc bag. Add lamb chops and toss to coat. Let the lamb chops marinate for 30 minutes at room temperature or up to 4 hours in the refrigerator.
2. Heat the broiler.
3. Remove lamb chops from marinade and pat dry with a paper towel. Season with salt and pepper. Place the chops in a flat layer on a broiler pan. Cook until medium rare and brown on the outside, approximately 2 to 3 minutes per side. (Alternatively, the chops can be grilled.)

SERVES 4

**THE F-FACTOR DIET NUTRITIONAL CONTENT FOR JOURNALING**
Per Serving: 0 g carbohydrate • 0 g fiber

**ACTUAL NUTRITIONAL CONTENT**
Per Serving: 254 calories • 0 g carbohydrate • 0 g fiber • 35 g protein • 12 g total fat • 4 g sat. fat • 148 mg sodium

# Grilled Veal Parmigiana

*I love veal parmigiana. But the customary recipe calls for breading and frying the cutlets—a no-no if you're trying to eat healthfully. This grilled version offers the same flavors without the extra fat and calories.*

4 4-ounce boneless veal cutlets
salt and pepper
1 teaspoon garlic powder
1 teaspoon dried oregano
½ cup prepared marinara sauce
1 cup shredded part-skim mozzarella cheese

1. Place veal cutlets in between 2 sheets of plastic wrap and flatten with a meat mallet until ¼-inch thick.
2. Season both sides of the cutlets with salt, pepper, garlic powder, and oregano.
3. Preheat the broiler. Heat a grill pan and grill cutlets 3 minutes on each side. Remove from the grill and place on a baking sheet.
4. Add 1 tablespoon marinara sauce to each cutlet and top with ¼ cup shredded cheese. Place under the broiler and cook until cheese is bubbly and begins to brown. Serve immediately.

SERVES 4

**THE F-FACTOR DIET NUTRITIONAL CONTENT FOR JOURNALING**
Per Serving: 0 g carbohydrate • 1 g fiber

**ACTUAL NUTRITIONAL CONTENT**
Per Serving: 362 calories • 3 g carbohydrate • 0 g fiber • 51 g protein • 15 g total fat • 7 g sat. fat • 737 mg sodium

## ✳ FISH AND SHELLFISH MAIN DISHES

# Shrimp with Feta Cheese

STEPS 1, 2, AND 3

*One of my favorite Greek restaurants in Manhattan, Meltemi, serves a dish just like this. My version is creamy, savory, and delicious, like the original.*

1 small onion, chopped
¼ cup white wine

1 14-ounce can diced tomatoes in liquid

2 tablespoons fresh parsley, chopped

½ teaspoon dried oregano

¼ teaspoon red pepper flakes

¼ teaspoon salt

16-ounce bag baby spinach

1¼ pounds medium/large shrimp, peeled and deveined

2 ounces feta cheese, crumbled

2 tablespoons fresh basil, chopped

1. In a large saucepan, cook the onion in the wine until the onion is translucent. Add the tomatoes and liquid, the parsley, oregano, red pepper, and salt, and cook on low heat for 12 minutes.
2. Add half the bag of baby spinach and stir to combine.
3. Add the shrimp and cook until they turn pink, about 2 to 3 minutes. Add the remaining spinach, and stir in the cheese and let it melt. Sprinkle with fresh basil and serve.

SERVES 4

**THE F-FACTOR DIET NUTRITIONAL CONTENT FOR JOURNALING**
Per Serving: 0 g carbohydrate • 4 g fiber

**ACTUAL NUTRITIONAL CONTENT**
Per Serving: 247 calories • 13 g carbohydrate • 4 g fiber • 34 g protein • 6 g total fat • 3 g sat. fat • 790 mg sodium

# Crispy Tilapia

STEPS 1, 2, AND 3

*You can often find crispy tilapia on a menu deep-fried. Mine is baked, and I have to say, I prefer my version every time.*

1 tablespoon light/low-fat mayonnaise

1 tablespoon mustard

3 6-ounce raw boneless, skinless tilapia fillets

3 GG Bran Crispbreads, pulverized into sprinkles
1 teaspoon garlic powder
1 teaspoon onion powder
1 teaspoon Italian seasoning
½ teaspoon paprika
½ teaspoon cayenne
1 teaspoon salt
½ teaspoon black pepper
nonstick cooking oil

1. Preheat oven to 425°F.
2. Mix the mayonnaise with the mustard and then coat each side of the tilapia with the mixture.
3. In a separate bowl, combine the remaining dry ingredients and use to completely coat each side of the tilapia fillets.
4. Spray a shallow baking dish with nonstick cooking spray. Lay the fillets flat in the dish, tucking thinner edges or ends under for more even cooking.
5. Bake in the preheated oven for 15 minutes, or until fish flakes easily with a fork.

SERVES 3

**THE F-FACTOR DIET NUTRITIONAL CONTENT FOR JOURNALING**
Per Serving: 9 g carbohydrate • 5 g fiber

ACTUAL NUTRITIONAL CONTENT
Per Serving: 155 calories • 9 g carbohydrate • 5 g fiber • 25 g protein • 3 g fat • 1 g sat. fat • 719 mg sodium

# Broiled Salmon with Dill

STEPS 1, 2, AND 3

*Although fish is often thought of as a "brain food," the latest findings say the real benefit is a healthy heart. Salmon is rich in omega-3 fatty acids, which reduce the risk of cardiovascular disease.*

1 onion, sliced
1 pound salmon fillet, cut into 4 pieces
salt and pepper
1 tablespoon olive oil
1½ tablespoon lemon juice
1 tablespoon chopped dill
1 lemon, cut into wedges

1. Preheat the broiler.
2. Place onion slices on the bottom of a broiler pan and place the salmon on top, skin side down.
3. Season the fish with salt and pepper. Sprinkle the olive oil, lemon juice, and dill on top.
4. Broil for 12 to 15 minutes, or until the fish is opaque.
5. Serve with lemon wedges.

SERVES 4

**THE F-FACTOR DIET NUTRITIONAL CONTENT FOR JOURNALING**
Per Serving: 0 g carbohydrate • 0 g fiber

**ACTUAL NUTRITIONAL CONTENT**
Per Serving: 173 calories • 3 g carbohydrate • 0 g fiber • 23 g protein • 7 g total fat • 1 g sat. fat • 115 mg sodium

## Asian-Flavored Tuna

STEPS 1, 2, AND 3

*While teriyaki sauce is tasty, it is also high in sugars. This recipe offers Asian flavors without the cloying sweetness of a typical teriyaki dish.*

4 tablespoons black peppercorns
4 4-ounce tuna steaks
2 tablespoons low-sodium soy sauce
2 tablespoons lemon juice
1 teaspoon minced ginger

2 tablespoons chicken stock
1 tablespoon chopped scallions
1 teaspoon minced garlic
4 whole scallions
nonstick cooking spray

1. Grind peppercorns on coarsest setting; place on a plate. Coat the tops and bottoms of the tuna steaks with the peppercorns. Set aside.
2. Combine soy sauce, lemon juice, ginger, and chicken stock in a saucepan. Bring to a boil. Add scallions and garlic and reduce heat to low. Keep warm.
3. Heat a grill pan and spray with nonstick spray. When pan is smoking, set the tuna steaks and whole scallions in pan and sear for 1½ minutes on each side (for rare tuna steaks).
4. Place tuna steaks on plates and serve with sauce. Garnish with the grilled whole scallions.

SERVES 4

**THE F-FACTOR DIET NUTRITIONAL CONTENT FOR JOURNALING**
Per Serving: 0 g carbohydrate • 0 g fiber

**ACTUAL NUTRITIONAL CONTENT**
Per Serving: 137 calories • 3 g carbohydrate • 0 g fiber • 28 g protein • 1 g total fat • 0 g sat. fat • 367 mg sodium

# Maryland Crab Cakes

STEPS 1, 2, AND 3

*Real Maryland crab cakes are all about the pure indulgence of crab, with as little filler and breading as possible. These cakes are delicious and easy to prepare.*

1 pound jumbo lump crabmeat, drained, and shell pieces removed
2 tablespoons 0% fat Greek yogurt
2 eggs (beaten)
1 teaspoon lime juice
2 tablespoons chopped cilantro

2 tablespoons chopped scallions
½ teaspoon chili powder
½ teaspoon cumin
nonstick cooking spray

1. Place crabmeat in a large mixing bowl. Set aside.
2. In a small mixing bowl, whisk together all remaining ingredients.
3. Add yogurt mixture to crabmeat and combine. Place mixture in a strainer set inside a large mixing bowl. Cover and refrigerate for minimum 1 hour, up to overnight (the longer, the better, as it will make crab cakes easier to form).
4. When ready to make crab cakes, remove from refrigerator, give mixture a good squeeze, and discard the liquid in the bowl.
5. Shape crab mixture into 6 cakes, squeezing out any excess liquid.
6. Coat a large cast-iron pan with nonstick cooking spray and place over medium-high heat. Cook crab cakes for 3 to 4 minutes on each side, until heated through and lightly browned. Repeat until all crab cakes are cooked. Serve warm.

SERVES 6

**THE F-FACTOR DIET NUTRITIONAL CONTENT FOR JOURNALING**
Per Serving: 0 g carbohydrate • 0 g fiber

**ACTUAL NUTRITIONAL CONTENT**
Per Serving: 97 calories • 1 g carbohydrate • 0 g fiber • 17 g protein • 3 g fat • 1 g sat. fat • 440 mg sodium

✳ SWEETS

# Vanilla-Bean Applesauce

STEPS 1, 2, AND 3

*Sweet tooth aching? This recipe is a delicious alternative to sugar-laden jellies and fruit compotes. The girls in the office love it on high-fiber crackers with cottage cheese, and it's great with the high-fiber pancakes, too.*

10–15 apples
1 vanilla bean (split lengthwise)
¼ cup water

1. Peel, core, and quarter 10–15 apples.
2. Add apples, vanilla bean, and water to a large pot on the stove. Place over high heat and bring to a boil.
3. Reduce the heat to medium, cover, and cook for 35–50 minutes without stirring. (The water will prevent the apples from scorching.)
4. Test for doneness by piercing apples with a fork—when they are very soft and almost falling apart, they're done. Remove from heat.
5. Remove the vanilla bean and allow to cool for a few minutes. Then, using the tip of a sharp knife, scrape the seeds into the pot and discard the pod.
6. Let apple mixture cook for another 5 minutes. Depending on your desired texture, use a food processor or potato masher to mash the fruit to your desired consistency.
7. Let applesauce cool completely, then transfer to one or more glass jars—applesauce will keep in fridge for up to 2 weeks.

SERVES 16

**THE F-FACTOR DIET NUTRITIONAL CONTENT FOR JOURNALING**
Per Serving: 17 g carbohydrate • 3 g fiber

**ACTUAL NUTRITIONAL CONTENT**
Per Serving: 71 calories • 17 g carbohydrate • 3 g fiber • 0 g protein • 0 g fat • 0 g sat. fat • 25 mg sodium

# Macerated Fruit

STEPS 1, 2, AND 3

*In college, I lived abroad in Florence with an Italian family. I never understood why the fruit salad tasted so good, until one day I asked my Italian "mom." She said the trick was to toss the fruit in fresh lemon juice and sugar. It not only gives it a bright flavor but the lemon helps to preserve the fruit so it doesn't spoil quickly.*

1 cup strawberries, sliced

1 cup blueberries

1 cup blackberries

1 mango, peeled and cubed

2 kiwis, peeled and sliced

1 lemon

2 tablespoons Truvia

1. Mix all the fruit together in a large bowl.
2. Cut lemon in half and squeeze juice over the fruit. Sprinkle on the Truvia and toss gently to coat. Chill and serve.

SERVES 6

**THE F-FACTOR DIET NUTRITIONAL CONTENT FOR JOURNALING**
Per Serving: 19 g carbohydrate • 4 g fiber

**ACTUAL NUTRITIONAL CONTENT**
Per Serving: 74 calories • 19 g carbohydrate • 4 g fiber • 1 g protein • 0 g total fat • 0 g sat. fat • 4 mg sodium

## Cheesecake Parfait with Blackberry Sauce

STEPS 1, 2, AND 3

*I love cheesecake but at more than 500 calories a slice, it's an infrequent indulgence. This recipe will satisfy your craving for the creamy taste of cheesecake—at a fraction of the fat and calories!*

½ cup low-fat ricotta cheese

4 ounces fat-free cream cheese

4 tablespoons Truvia

1 teaspoon vanilla extract

2 cups raspberries (leave a few aside for garnish)

2 cups blackberries

2 tablespoons water

1. In a blender or food processor, combine the ricotta cheese, cream cheese, 2 tablespoons of the sweetener, vanilla, and raspberries. Process until smooth. Transfer to a bowl.
2. Rinse out blender or food processor; add blackberries, water, and the remaining 2 tablespoons sweetener. Pulse to chop blackberries.
3. Using half of the raspberry-cheese mixture, divide among 4 dessert goblets. Top with half of the blackberry sauce. Add remaining raspberry mixture and top with remaining sauce. Sprinkle with remaining raspberries. Chill for at least an hour in the refrigerator.

SERVES 4

**THE F-FACTOR DIET NUTRITIONAL CONTENT FOR JOURNALING**
Per Serving: 20 g carbohydrate • 8 g fiber

**ACTUAL NUTRITIONAL CONTENT**
Per Serving: 137 calories • 20 g carbohydrate • 8 g fiber • 8 g protein • 3 g total fat • 2 g sat. fat • 193 mg sodium

## Grilled Fruit Kebabs

STEPS 1, 2, AND 3

*These are great in the summer, especially at the end of a barbecue dinner.*

4 bamboo skewers
1 teaspoon canola oil
8 large strawberries
1 peach, quartered
2 apricots, halved
1 plum, quartered

1. Soak skewers in cold water for 30 minutes.
2. Heat a grill pan on medium-high heat. Brush with canola oil.
3. Thread the fruit on the skewers beginning with a strawberry, then a quarter of a peach, half an apricot, a quarter of a plum, and topped with another strawberry. Repeat for the three remaining skewers.

4. Grill the kebabs, turning once, until lightly browned and softened, about 5 minutes.

SERVES 4

**THE F-FACTOR DIET NUTRITIONAL CONTENT FOR JOURNALING**
Per Serving: 9 g carbohydrate • 2 g fiber

**ACTUAL NUTRITIONAL CONTENT**
Per Serving: 49 calories • 9 g carbohydrate • 2 g fiber • 1 g protein • 2 g total fat • 0 g sat. fat • 1 mg sodium

✳ BREAKFAST FOODS

# Chunky Monkey F-Factor Smoothie

STEPS 2 AND 3

*Chocolate, banana, and peanut butter . . . Need I say more? Best part about this chunky monkey smoothie is that it will leave you feeling full—and far from chunky!*

> 1 cup crushed ice
> ½ cup unsweetened almond milk
> 2 tablespoon PB2 powdered peanut butter
> 2 scoops F-Factor Chocolate Fiber/Protein Powder
> ½ frozen banana, sliced

Combine all ingredients in a blender. Cover and blend to desired consistency.

SERVES 1

**THE F-FACTOR DIET NUTRITIONAL CONTENT FOR JOURNALING**
Per Serving: 44 g carbohydrate • 24 g fiber

**ACTUAL NUTRITIONAL CONTENT**
Per Serving: 246 calories • 53 g carbohydrate • 24 g fiber • 26 g protein • 5 g fat • 0 sat. fat • 165 mg sodium

# Pumpkin Spice Overnight Oats

STEPS 2 AND 3

*Make before bed, eat before work. This easier-than-easy recipe is OAT-of-this-world delicious and, with its combination of fiber and protein, will keep you feeling (fiber)FULL till lunch, for sure.*

½ cup rolled oats

1 cup unsweetened vanilla almond milk

2 scoops F-Factor Vanilla Fiber/Protein Powder

1 tablespoon pumpkin pie spice

½ teaspoon cinnamon

½ teaspoon nutmeg

1. In a mason jar, combine all the ingredients. Place lid on loosely and place in refrigerator overnight.
2. In the morning, remove from refrigerator, stir (mixing well), and enjoy. If it appears too dry, you can give it a splash more of almond milk.

SERVES 2

**THE F-FACTOR DIET NUTRITIONAL CONTENT FOR JOURNALING**
Per Serving: 28 g carbohydrate • 14 g fiber

**ACTUAL NUTRITIONAL CONTENT**
Per Serving: 166 calories • 30 g carbohydrate • 14 g fiber • 14 g protein • 4 g fat • 1 g sat. fat • 38 mg sodium

## Breakfast Burritos

STEPS 2 AND 3

*This is a filling and tasty brunch dish that is perfect to make when you have guests.*

8 eggs

3 scallions, chopped

1 4-ounce can green chilies, drained and chopped

1 small tomato, diced

salt and pepper

½ cup grated cheddar cheese

2 tablespoons cilantro, chopped

4 La Tortilla Factory low-carb/low-fat large tortillas

nonstick cooking spray

1. Beat 4 whole eggs and 4 additional egg whites in a shallow bowl (discard 4 yolks).
2. Spray a medium nonstick skillet with cooking spray and heat over medium heat. Add the scallions, chilies, and tomato. Season with salt and pepper. Sauté for 3 minutes.
3. Add the beaten eggs to the skillet and continue to stir and cook until the eggs are fully set. Remove from heat and stir in cheddar cheese and cilantro.
4. Place tortillas between two damp paper towels and microwave for 20 seconds. This makes them softer and easier to roll up.
5. Divide egg mixture among the tortillas and roll up.

SERVES 4

**THE F-FACTOR DIET NUTRITIONAL CONTENT FOR JOURNALING**
Per Serving: 14 g carbohydrate • 15 g fiber

**ACTUAL NUTRITIONAL CONTENT**
Per Serving: 233 calories • 22 g carbohydrate • 15 g fiber • 21 g protein • 13 g total fat • 4 g sat. fat • 773 mg sodium

# Banana Chocolate Chip Muffins

STEPS 2 AND 3

*These are B-A-N-A-N-A-S! A typical store-bought muffin can deliver close to 500 calories and no fiber. These muffins are less than 200 calories each, and they pack in 9 grams of the good stuff.*

nonstick cooking spray
1 medium banana
1 cup 0% fat plain Greek yogurt
2 eggs
1 tablespoon vanilla extract
½ cup oats
8 GG Bran Crispbreads, pulverized into sprinkles
1 tablespoon Truvia
sprinkle of salt

½ teaspoon baking soda

1½ teaspoons baking powder

¼ cup Lily's Dark Chocolate Premium Baking Chips

1. Preheat oven to 400°F. Coat either a 6-cup or 12-cup muffin tray (depending on desired muffin size) with nonstick cooking spray and set aside.

2. In a large bowl, mash banana. Add yogurt, eggs, and vanilla extract. Mix well.

3. Fold in oats, GG sprinkles, Truvia, salt, baking soda, baking powder, and chocolate chips to the wet ingredients.

4. Divide batter among prepared muffin cups, filling each about ¾ full.

5. Bake approximately 15 minutes, until muffin tops are pale gold and tester inserted into center comes out with some melted chocolate chips attached but no crumbs.

6. Transfer muffins to cooling rack.

SERVES 6 (1 LARGE MUFFIN OR 2 MINI MUFFINS PER SERVING)

**THE F-FACTOR DIET NUTRITIONAL CONTENT FOR JOURNALING**
Per Serving: 26 g carbohydrate • 9 g fiber

**ACTUAL NUTRITIONAL CONTENT**
Per Serving: 165 calories • 27 g carbohydrate • 9 g fiber • 9 g protein • 5 g fat • 2 g sat. fat • 259 mg sodium

## Italian Herb Frittata

STEPS 2 AND 3

*The colors of the Italian flag are represented in this omelet: red (tomato), white (onion), and green (spinach).*

nonstick cooking spray

3 egg whites

¼ cup low-fat cottage cheese

1 tablespoon grated Parmesan cheese

2 tablespoons cold water

¼ teaspoon dried basil

¼ teaspoon dried oregano

2 tablespoons diced onion

½ cup frozen spinach, defrosted and squeezed dry

1 plum tomato, diced

salt and pepper

1. In a bowl, whisk together egg whites, cottage cheese, Parmesan cheese, water, basil, and oregano. Set aside.
2. Heat a nonstick pan with cooking spray. Add onion and cook for 2 minutes. Add spinach and tomato and cook for 2 minutes more. Season with salt and pepper.
3. Add the spinach mixture to the egg mixture.
4. Spray the pan with nonstick spray and pour the egg-vegetable mixture back into the pan. Cover and cook for 5 minutes. Turn over onto a plate and serve.

SERVES 1

**THE F-FACTOR DIET NUTRITIONAL CONTENT FOR JOURNALING**
Per Serving: 0 g carbohydrate • 4 g fiber

**ACTUAL NUTRITIONAL CONTENT**
Per Serving: 162 calories • 11 g carbohydrate • 4 g fiber • 23 g protein • 3 g total fat • 2 g sat. fat • 551 mg sodium

## The F-Factor Breakfast Sandwich

STEPS 2 AND 3

*This is my take on McDonald's Egg McMuffin. This version has more fiber and fewer grams of fat. I promise, you won't miss a thing!*

nonstick cooking spray

1 slice Canadian bacon

1 egg

1 slice Kraft Free American cheese

1 Thomas' light multigrain English muffin

1. In a nonstick skillet, cook Canadian bacon until lightly browned on both sides. Remove from pan and set aside.
2. Spray pan with nonstick spray. Add egg and scramble.
3. While egg is cooking, place half the cheese on one half of the English muffin and put both sides into a toaster oven to toast.
4. Remove English muffin from toaster oven, place Canadian bacon and scrambled egg on muffin, and top with the side with the remaining cheese. Enjoy!

SERVES 1

**THE F-FACTOR DIET NUTRITIONAL CONTENT FOR JOURNALING**
Per Serving: 22 g carbohydrate • 8 g fiber

**ACTUAL NUTRITIONAL CONTENT**
Per Serving: 248 calories • 28 g carbohydrate • 8 g fiber • 21 g protein • 7 g total fat • 2 g sat. fat • 861 mg sodium

## ✳ SOUPS, SALADS, AND VEGETABLES

# Moroccan Lentil Soup

STEPS 2 AND 3

*I'm a soup fanatic. Homemade soups, like this one, are a great opportunity to fill up on a nutritious blend of vegetables, beans, and lean protein. This soup actually tastes better the second day, when the flavors have had a chance to develop.*

cooking spray
1 medium onion, chopped
1 cup carrots, chopped
1 cup celery, chopped
1 cup mushrooms, sliced
8 ounces chicken tenders, cut into bite-sized pieces
1 cup brown lentils
1 14.5-ounce can garbanzo beans, rinsed and drained
1 14.5-ounce can chopped tomatoes
3 cups chicken broth

2 cups water

2 teaspoons cumin

1 teaspoon oregano

1 teaspoon Kosher salt

¼ teaspoon black pepper

1. Coat a large pot with cooking spray and heat on high heat. Sauté the onion until soft. Add the carrots, celery, mushrooms, and chicken. Sauté for
   a few minutes, until chicken is lightly browned.
2. Add lentils, garbanzo beans, tomatoes, chicken broth, water, herbs, salt,
   and pepper. Bring to a boil. Cover, reduce heat, and simmer for 1 hour.

SERVES 12

**THE F-FACTOR DIET NUTRITIONAL CONTENT FOR JOURNALING**
Per Serving: 15 g carbohydrate • 8 g fiber

**ACTUAL NUTRITIONAL CONTENT**
Per Serving: 145 calories • 22 g carbohydrate • 8 g fiber • 13 g protein • 1 g total fat • 0 g sat.
fat • 591 mg sodium

## Black Bean Soup

STEPS 2 AND 3

*Puréeing gives this soup a wonderful consistency that will hold up to all the deli-
cious toppings you can add. I love topping it with diced onion, chopped cilantro,
and a wedge of lime.*

nonstick cooking spray

3 cloves garlic, minced

1 onion, chopped

2 cups water

3 cups chicken broth

1 cup carrots, chopped

1 cup celery, chopped

1 green bell pepper, seeded and chopped

8 ounces chicken breast, cubed

1 cup canned black beans, rinsed

1 teaspoon dried oregano

1 teaspoon cumin

1 teaspoon Kosher salt

¼ teaspoon black pepper

OPTIONAL TOPPINGS:

nonfat sour cream

lime wedges

chopped onion

chopped tomato

chopped cilantro

low-fat cheddar cheese

1. Coat a large stockpot with nonstick cooking spray and heat over high heat. Sauté garlic and onion until soft, approximately 3 minutes.
2. Add the remaining ingredients, stir, and bring to a boil.
3. Cover, reduce heat to medium, and cook for 2 hours, stirring occasionally.
4. Place ½ of soup mixture into a blender and blend. Return the blended soup to the stockpot and stir to combine.
5. Place in bowl and serve with optional toppings.

SERVES 8

**THE F-FACTOR DIET NUTRITIONAL CONTENT FOR JOURNALING**
Per Serving: 10 g carbohydrate • 5 g fiber

**ACTUAL NUTRITIONAL CONTENT**
Per Serving: 134 calories • 20 g carbohydrate • 5 g fiber • 12 g protein • 1 g total fat • 0 g sat. fat • 330 mg sodium

# Minestrone Soup

STEPS 2 AND 3

*I've skipped the usual pasta and added fiber-rich barley instead. Barley has a chewy texture and nutty taste that adds body and flavor.*

nonstick cooking spray

2 cloves garlic

1 onion, chopped

1 cup carrots, chopped

1 cup celery, chopped

2 zucchini, diced

2 cups mushrooms, sliced

1 14.5-ounce can cannellini beans

1 14.5-ounce can chopped tomatoes

½ cup barley

1 teaspoon oregano

1 teaspoon basil

1 teaspoon Kosher salt

4 teaspoons black pepper

5 cups chicken broth or vegetable broth

2 cups fresh spinach, chopped

8 tablespoons grated Parmesan cheese

1. Spray a large pot with nonstick cooking spray and heat over high heat. Add garlic and onion and sauté until the onion is soft.
2. Add the carrots, celery, zucchini, mushrooms, beans, chopped tomatoes, barley, seasonings, and broth.
3. Bring to a boil. Cover and reduce heat. Simmer for 1 hour. Right before serving, add the spinach and stir until it wilts.
4. Serve and top with a tablespoon of grated Parmesan cheese.

SERVES 8

**THE F-FACTOR DIET NUTRITIONAL CONTENT FOR JOURNALING**
Per Serving: 13 g carbohydrate • 8 g fiber

**ACTUAL NUTRITIONAL CONTENT**
Per Serving: 195 calories • 31 g carbohydrate • 8 g fiber • 13 g protein • 3 g total fat • 0 g sat. fat • 1259 mg sodium

RECIPES

# Tanya's House Salad

*This salad is a staple in my home—I make it at the beginning of every week. There isn't much to do besides rinsing, chopping, and can opening. The salad is so big that it lasts for days, and I have salad on hand whenever I'm in the mood for it.*

1 bag romaine hearts (3 hearts)
1 bag baby carrots
2 celery hearts
1 red pepper
1 seedless cucumber
1 box cherry tomatoes
1 14-ounce can hearts of palm
1 14-ounce can garbanzo beans
1 red onion

1. Chop the lettuce and place it at the bottom of the bowl.
2. Next, chop the carrots and celery into bite-sized pieces and layer on top of lettuce.
3. Seed and chop the red pepper. Add to salad.
4. Peel cucumber, cut in half lengthwise, and then into ¼-inch slices. Add to salad.
5. Rinse tomatoes, dry, and add to the salad.
6. Drain the hearts of palm, chop, and add to salad.
7. Rinse garbanzo beans in a colander and add to salad.
8. Halve the onion and slice thin. Add to salad.
9. Serve.

SERVES 8

**THE F-FACTOR DIET NUTRITIONAL CONTENT FOR JOURNALING**
Per Serving: 6 g carbohydrate • 8 g fiber

**ACTUAL NUTRITIONAL CONTENT**
Per Serving: 147 calories • 26 g carbohydrate • 8 g fiber • 8 g protein • 2 g total fat • 0 g sat. fat • 288 mg sodium

RECIPES

# Asian Chicken Salad

*I make this salad whenever I invite my girlfriends over. It's light yet filling, and everyone walks away from the table happy.*

DRESSING INGREDIENTS:

3 tablespoons seasoned rice vinegar

2 tablespoons low-sodium soy sauce

1½ tablespoons dark sesame oil

1 clove garlic, minced

½ teaspoon minced fresh ginger

½ teaspoon sugar

SALAD INGREDIENTS:

3 cups baby spinach

4 cups napa cabbage, shredded

2 cups shredded rotisserie chicken, breast meat only

½ cup snow peas, cut lengthwise into three strips each

½ cup julienned carrots (packaged)

½ cup scallions, diagonally sliced

¼ cup chopped cilantro

2 teaspoons sesame seeds, toasted

1. Combine all the dressing ingredients in a blender. Blend to combine. Set aside.
2. Combine the salad ingredients in a large bowl. Pour dressing over salad. Toss well and serve.

SERVES 4

**THE F-FACTOR DIET NUTRITIONAL CONTENT FOR JOURNALING**
Per Serving: 0 g carbohydrate • 3 g fiber

**ACTUAL NUTRITIONAL CONTENT**
Per Serving: 212 calories • 8 g carbohydrate • 3 g fiber • 25 g protein • 9 g total fat • 2 g sat. fat • 588 mg sodium

# Lettuce-less Greek Salad

*Switch it up by swapping it out! This play on a traditional Greek salad presents well and tastes delicious. Opa!*

DRESSING INGREDIENTS:

4 tablespoons olive oil

2 tablespoons fresh lemon juice

½ teaspoon fresh chopped garlic

1 teaspoon red wine vinegar

½ teaspoon dried oregano

½ teaspoon dried dill weed

salt and pepper

SALAD INGREDIENTS:

3 large cucumbers (should yield 5 cups when spiralized)

3 large plum tomatoes, seeded, coarsely chopped

⅓ red onion, peeled, chopped

1 green bell pepper, seeded, coarsely chopped

½ cup pitted black olives, coarsely chopped

1 cup crumbled feta cheese

1. Prepare dressing by whisking the olive oil, lemon juice, garlic, vinegar, oregano, and dill weed until well blended. Season to taste with salt and pepper.
2. Spiralize cucumber using a spiralizer, mandoline, or peeler. Cut cucumber strands occasionally to create smaller, easier-to-eat pieces. (If you don't have a spiralizer, you can just peel and cube cucumbers.) Place in salad bowl.
3. Combine remaining salad ingredients, minus the cheese. Toss with dressing.
4. Sprinkle cheese over the top and serve.

**THE F-FACTOR DIET NUTRITIONAL CONTENT FOR JOURNALING**
Per Serving: 2 g carbohydrate • 3 g fiber

**ACTUAL NUTRITIONAL CONTENT**
Per Serving: 204 calories • 11 g carbohydrate • 3 g fiber • 6 g protein • 16 g fat • 5 g sat. fat •
346 mg sodium

# Roasted Corn Salsa

STEPS 2 AND 3

*Winter, spring, summer, or fall, with this dish you can have it all. It is a perfect
salad or side, and a great addition to your Taco Tuesdays.*

  1 16-ounce bag frozen sweet corn
  3 pinches of salt (1 for cooking the corn and the rest for when all
    ingredients are added)
  ¼ red bell pepper, finely chopped
  ¼ red onion, finely chopped
  seeds from 1 jalapeño, to taste
  juice from ½ lime
  cilantro, to taste

1. Add corn to a nonstick pan over high heat with a pinch of salt and roast
   for 10 minutes.
2. Transfer to a large bowl and cool.
3. Combine chopped red bell pepper, onion, jalapeño, lime juice, cilantro,
   and remaining salt in a separate bowl.
4. Once corn has chilled, combine with the remaining ingredients.
5. Serve chilled.

SERVES 4

**THE F-FACTOR DIET NUTRITIONAL CONTENT FOR JOURNALING**
Per Serving: 15 g carbohydrate • 3 g fiber

Per Serving: 70 calories • 16 g carbohydrate • 3 g fiber • 2 g protein • 1 g fat • 0 g sat. fat • 119 mg sodium

## Cauliflower "Fried Rice"

STEPS 2 AND 3

*Comfort food and healthy food don't have to be mutually exclusive. Rather than ordering carb-heavy, sodium-laden fried rice takeout, whip up your own in less than 20 minutes! Fast, easy, delicious, and nutritious—your skinny jeans will thank you.*

> 3 cups of grated raw cauliflower (purchase riced cauliflower or use a cheese grater or food processor to rice)
> 2 teaspoons olive oil
> 3–4 garlic cloves, minced
> ½ cup onion, diced
> ½ cup frozen peas
> ½ cup carrots, thinly sliced
> 2 eggs (or 4 egg whites), scrambled
> 3 tablespoons low-sodium soy sauce

1. If not using pre-riced cauliflower, wash and rice/grate cauliflower head and set aside.
2. In a large pan over medium-high heat, sauté garlic and onions in olive oil, until onions become soft and transparent (about 2 to 3 minutes).
3. Add peas and carrots to the pan and cook until carrots begin to soften and peas are heated through (about 3 to 4 minutes).
4. Stir in scrambled eggs, riced cauliflower, and soy sauce.
5. Cook, stirring frequently, for about 5 to 7 more minutes.
6. Remove from heat and serve.

SERVES 4

**THE F-FACTOR DIET NUTRITIONAL CONTENT FOR JOURNALING**
Per Serving: 4 g carbohydrate • 5 g fiber

# Sweet Potato Chips

*These chips have all the crunch of regular potato chips without all the fat. Sweet
potatoes are also a great source of vitamin A and antioxidants—so dig in!*

**nonstick cooking spray**
**½ pound sweet potatoes**
**½ tablespoon canola oil**
**¼ teaspoon Kosher salt**

1. Preheat oven to 400°F. Lightly coat a baking sheet with nonstick cooking
   spray.
2. Slice the sweet potatoes into very thin slices.
3. In a large bowl, toss potatoes with canola oil and salt to coat the chips
   lightly. Lay the slices in a single layer on the prepared baking sheet.
4. Bake for 15 minutes. Turn over each chip and bake for 5 minutes more.
   Chips should be crisp. If not, bake up to 3 more minutes, checking every
   minute so the chips won't burn. Let cool before serving.

SERVES 4 (APPROXIMATELY 15 CHIPS EACH)

**THE F-FACTOR DIET NUTRITIONAL CONTENT FOR JOURNALING**
Per Serving: 14 g carbohydrate • 2 g fiber

**ACTUAL NUTRITIONAL CONTENT**
Per Serving: 75 calories • 14 g carbohydrate • 2 g fiber • 1 g protein • 2 g total fat • 0 g sat.
fat • 153 mg sodium

# Spiced Garbanzo Beans

*The Standard Hotel in Miami serves a snack similar to this one at poolside. They are delicious as a snack or as a side for roasted fish.*

nonstick cooking spray
2 15.5-ounce cans garbanzo beans
2 tablespoons cumin
1 tablespoon curry powder
1 teaspoon chili powder
½ teaspoon salt
⅛ teaspoon pepper

1. Preheat oven to 350°F.
2. Drain garbanzo beans and place in a bowl.
3. Add the rest of the ingredients and toss well to coat.
4. Spray a baking sheet with nonstick cooking spray. Spread garbanzo beans out in a layer and bake in oven for 15 minutes, stirring halfway through.
5. Place in a bowl and serve warm.

SERVES 8

**THE F-FACTOR DIET NUTRITIONAL CONTENT FOR JOURNALING**
Per Serving: 33 g carbohydrate • 8 g fiber

**ACTUAL NUTRITIONAL CONTENT**
Per Serving: 198 calories • 33 g carbohydrate • 8 g fiber • 11 g protein • 3 g total fat • 0 g sat. fat • 267 mg sodium

✳ CHICKEN AND TURKEY MAIN DISHES

# Scallion and Ginger Spiced Chicken

*This chicken is wonderful served with sautéed spinach and brown rice.*

4 4-ounce boneless, skinless chicken breasts
salt and pepper
1 teaspoon sesame oil
¼ cup minced scallions, white part only
3 cloves garlic, minced
1 tablespoon fresh ginger, minced
1 cup reduced-sodium chicken broth
¾ cup rice wine vinegar
2 tablespoons hoisin sauce
2 teaspoons sugar
1 tablespoon low-sodium soy sauce
1 cup shelled edamame, defrosted
½ cup sliced scallions, green part only

1. Season chicken breast with salt and pepper. Spray a nonstick skillet with cooking spray and heat over high heat. Add the chicken and sear until well browned on both sides, about 3 minutes per side. Transfer chicken to a plate and tent with foil to keep warm.
2. Reduce the heat to medium and add the sesame oil. Add the minced scallion whites, garlic, and ginger. Cook, stirring 1 minute.
3. Add the chicken broth, vinegar, hoisin sauce, sugar, and soy sauce. Bring to a simmer. Cook until slightly thickened, about 3 minutes.
4. Return the chicken and juices to the skillet and reduce the heat to low. Add the edamame. Simmer until the chicken is cooked through, about 4 minutes.
5. Transfer the chicken to a platter and spoon the sauce over the chicken. Garnish with green scallions.

SERVES 4

**THE F-FACTOR DIET NUTRITIONAL CONTENT FOR JOURNALING**
Per Serving: 14 g carbohydrate • 3 g fiber

**ACTUAL NUTRITIONAL CONTENT**
Per Serving: 317 calories • 14 g carbohydrate • 3 g fiber • 44 g protein • 9 g total fat • 2 g sat. fat • 853 mg sodium

# Crispy Pecan Chicken

*The nutty coating on this chicken makes it satisfying. Who needs greasy fried chicken when you have this crispy, crunchy dish?*

> 4 4-ounce boneless, skinless chicken breasts
> 1 cup buttermilk or plain yogurt
> 1 cup All-Bran Original
> ⅓ cup finely chopped pecans
> 1 teaspoon lemon pepper
> ¾ teaspoon poultry seasoning
> ¼ teaspoon salt
> cooking spray

1. Place a chicken breast between 2 sheets of plastic wrap and flatten with a meat mallet to ½-inch thickness. Repeat with remaining breasts.
2. Place the chicken in a glass bowl and cover with the buttermilk. Turn the chicken to coat. Cover, and refrigerate for 6 to 24 hours, turning occasionally.
3. Put the cereal in a food processor and process into coarse crumbs. Alternatively, you can put the cereal in a resealable plastic bag and crush with a rolling pin or with your hands. You will have approximately 1 cup of crumbs. Put the crumbs in a shallow dish and add the pecans, lemon pepper, poultry seasoning, and salt. Stir to combine.
4. Remove the chicken from the buttermilk and shake off the excess. Dip the chicken in the cereal mixture, turning to coat both sides well.
5. Coat a baking sheet with cooking spray and arrange the chicken in a single layer. Coat the tops lightly with cooking spray and bake at 400°F for about 25 minutes, or until the chicken is crisp and gold on the outside and is cooked through. Serve hot.

SERVES 4

**THE F-FACTOR DIET NUTRITIONAL CONTENT FOR JOURNALING**
Per Serving: 17 g carbohydrate • 10 g fiber

**ACTUAL NUTRITIONAL CONTENT**

Per Serving: 300 calories • 17 g carbohydrate • 10 g fiber • 38 g protein • 10 g total fat • 2 g sat. fat • 574 mg sodium

## Chicken Ratatouille

STEPS 1, 2, AND 3

*This dish is incredibly versatile: use it as an omelet filling or a sauce for pasta, or serve it in a bowl as stew.*

    1 tablespoon olive oil
    1 cup onion, chopped
    2 cloves garlic, minced
    4 4-ounce boneless, skinless chicken breasts, cut into 1-inch pieces
    2 cups cubed eggplant (skin on)
    1 medium zucchini, halved and sliced
    1 cup sliced mushrooms
    1 cup chopped tomatoes
    1 8-ounce can tomato sauce
    1 tablespoon tomato paste
    ½ teaspoon dried oregano
    1 teaspoon dried basil
    ¼ teaspoon dried rosemary
    ¼ teaspoon dried fennel seeds
    salt and pepper

1. In a large skillet, heat olive oil and sauté onion and garlic until tender. Add the chicken and cook for 3 minutes, stirring frequently, until chicken is well browned. Stir in the vegetables, chopped tomatoes, tomato sauce, tomato paste, and dried herbs. Season with salt and pepper.
2. Bring mixture to a boil. Reduce heat; simmer, covered, for 20 minutes or till tender. Uncover and cook 5 to 10 minutes more, until sauce thickens, stirring occasionally.

RECIPES

SERVES 8

**THE F-FACTOR DIET NUTRITIONAL CONTENT FOR JOURNALING**
Per Serving: 0 g carbohydrate • 4 g fiber

**ACTUAL NUTRITIONAL CONTENT**
Per Serving: 143 calories • 8 g carbohydrate • 4 g fiber • 19 g protein • 4 g total fat • 1 g sat.
fat • 348 mg sodium

# Roasted Chicken Harvest Bowl

STEPS 2 AND 3

*Who said you can't enjoy fall flavors all year long? Served warm or cold, this dish
not only looks pretty but tastes great, too.*

1 8-ounce chicken breast
nonstick cooking spray
3 cups kale, leaves torn, stems chopped
1 cup butternut squash, cubed
1 yellow onion, diced
1 apple, cored and thinly sliced
2 cups shredded red cabbage
juice of 1 lemon
2 tablespoons apple cider vinegar
1 tablespoon Dijon mustard
1 teaspoon Truvia
2 tablespoons olive oil
salt and pepper to taste

1. Preheat oven to 350°F. Line a sheet pan with tinfoil.
2. Coat chicken breast with nonstick cooking spray, place atop prepared
   sheet pan, and roast in oven until chicken has cooked through, about 25
   minutes. Allow chicken to cool and shred meat. Set aside.
3. Chop kale, separating the kale stems from the leaves, and other vegetables
   and apple.

4. Coat a large pan with nonstick cooking spray and place over medium-high heat. Add kale stems, squash, and onion and cook until onions are translucent, about 5 minutes.

5. Add kale leaves, apple, cabbage, ¼ cup water, and juice from ½ a lemon to the pan. Mix well and cook until kale begins to wilt, about 5 minutes.

6. Remove from heat and add salt and pepper to taste. Add shredded chicken to the vegetables.

7. in a small bowl, whisk together apple cider vinegar, mustard, Truvia, the remaining lemon juice, and olive oil. Add salt and pepper to taste and spoon over warm salad.

SERVES 2

**THE F-FACTOR DIET NUTRITIONAL CONTENT FOR JOURNALING**
Per Serving: 21 g carbohydrate • 6 g fiber

**ACTUAL NUTRITIONAL CONTENT**
Per Serving: 368 calories • 35 g carbohydrate • 6 g fiber • 23 g protein • 17 g fat • 2 sat. fat • 1,321 mg sodium

# Turkey Chili

STEPS 2 AND 3

*When it's cold outside, there's nothing that warms my belly more than a big bowl of chili. And because this recipe contains fiber-rich beans, it really fills you up and keeps you satisfied.*

1 pound lean ground turkey
1 small onion, chopped
3 15-ounce cans red kidney beans, drained
3 14.5-ounce cans chopped tomatoes
1 cup water
2 celery stalks, chopped
1 medium green pepper, seeded and chopped
¼ cup red wine vinegar
2 tablespoons chili powder

2 teaspoons ground cumin
1 teaspoon dried oregano
1 teaspoon dried parsley
1 teaspoon dried basil

OPTIONAL TOPPINGS:
grated cheddar cheese
diced onion
low-fat sour cream

1. Heat a large stockpot over medium-high heat until hot. Add ground turkey and chopped onion and cook until browned.
2. Add the remaining ingredients and bring to a boil. Reduce heat and simmer on low heat for 2 hours.
3. Garnish with optional toppings if desired.

SERVES 8

**THE F-FACTOR DIET NUTRITIONAL CONTENT FOR JOURNALING**
Per Serving: 39 g carbohydrate • 13 g fiber

**ACTUAL NUTRITIONAL CONTENT**
Per Serving: 282 calories • 39 g carbohydrate • 13 g fiber • 20 g protein • 6 g total fat • 1 g sat. fat • 967 mg sodium

✳ BEEF, PORK, AND LAMB MAIN DISHES

# Easy Beef Fajitas

STEPS 2 AND 3

*Fajitas are one of the healthiest dishes to order at a Mexican restaurant. Here's an easy version to make at home.*

1 pound boneless beefsteak
2 tablespoons lime juice
1 garlic clove, minced
½ teaspoon chili powder

½ teaspoon dried oregano, crushed

4 La Tortilla Factory whole-wheat low-carb/low-fat tortillas

cooking spray

1 medium onion, sliced thin

1 medium red pepper, cut into thin strips

1 14.5-ounce can black beans, drained

½ cup chopped tomato

¼ cup salsa

½ cup shredded lettuce

¼ cup fat-free sour cream

1. Slice beef into thin strips. Toss with lime juice, garlic, chili powder, and oregano. Marinate for 1 hour and up to 24 hours.
2. Wrap tortillas in foil. Heat oven to 350°F and place tortillas in oven.
3. Spray a nonstick pan with cooking spray. Add onion and cook for 1½ minutes. Add red pepper and cook for 1½ minutes more. Remove vegetables from the skillet.
4. Add the beef strips and cook until desired doneness. Drain off any fat. Add black beans, tomato, and cooked onion and peppers.
5. Fill warm tortillas with beef mixture and top with salsa, lettuce, and sour cream. Serve immediately.

SERVES 4

**THE F-FACTOR DIET NUTRITIONAL CONTENT FOR JOURNALING**
Per Serving: 43 g carbohydrate • 4 g fiber

**ACTUAL NUTRITIONAL CONTENT**
Per Serving: 370 calories • 48 g carbohydrate • 8 g fiber • 21 g protein • 12 g total fat •
4 g sat. fat • 326 mg sodium

## Wholesome Sloppy Joes

STEPS 2 AND 3

*Growing up, I loved eating sloppy joes. I wanted to create the same flavors while boosting the fiber. Adding lentils did the trick—and you won't even notice they're in there! Serving on whole-wheat buns adds even more fiber.*

¾ pound lean ground beef

½ cup chopped onion

½ cup chopped green bell pepper

1 garlic clove, minced

1 8-ounce can tomato sauce

½ cup uncooked lentils

⅔ cup water

¼ cup ketchup

1 teaspoon red wine vinegar

½ teaspoon paprika

½ teaspoon salt

¼ teaspoon pepper

½ teaspoon dry mustard

4 whole-wheat sandwich buns

1. In a large skillet over medium-high heat, brown beef with onion, green pepper, and garlic. Drain well.
2. Stir in remaining ingredients except sandwich buns.
3. Reduce heat, cover, and simmer 40 to 45 minutes or until lentils are tender. Spoon ¼ of mixture onto each bun.

SERVES 4

**THE F-FACTOR DIET NUTRITIONAL CONTENT FOR JOURNALING**
Per Serving: 33 g carbohydrate • 7 g fiber

**ACTUAL NUTRITIONAL CONTENT**
Per Serving: 338 calories • 26 g carbohydrate • 9 g fiber • 24 g protein • 16 g total fat • 6 g sat. fat • 583 mg sodium

## Grilled Beef and Bean Burgers*

STEPS 2 AND 3

*These juicy burgers are so delicious that no one will guess they contain high-fiber beans.*

1 15.5-ounce can great northern beans, rinsed and drained

½ pound extra-lean ground beef

4 GG Bran Crispbreads, pulverized into sprinkles

2 tablespoons barbecue sauce

¼ teaspoon pepper

1 egg

5 whole-wheat hamburger buns

OPTIONAL TOPPINGS:

lettuce

tomato

sliced onion

1. Heat an outdoor grill or an indoor grill pan.
2. Place beans in a bowl and mash with a fork. Add the beef, sprinkles, barbecue sauce, pepper, and the egg. Mix well to combine and shape mixture into 5 patties, about ½ inch thick.
3. Grill the patties for about 5 minutes per side, or to desired doneness.
4. Serve on whole-wheat buns and top with lettuce, tomato, and onion.

SERVES 5

*Recipe courtesy of the U.S. Dried Bean Council.

**THE F-FACTOR DIET NUTRITIONAL CONTENT FOR JOURNALING**
Per Serving: 43 g carbohydrate • 9 g fiber

**ACTUAL NUTRITIONAL CONTENT**
Per Serving: 344 calories • 43 g carbohydrate • 9 g fiber • 20 g protein • 11 g total fat • 4 g sat. fat • 353 mg sodium

## Best Meat Loaf

STEPS 2 AND 3

*Everyone's mom seems to have a recipe for meat loaf. Now that I'm a mom, I figured it was time for me to come up with a recipe of my own. My meat loaf is so moist, no one notices it is made from lean ground beef. I think my mom would approve!*

**MEAT LOAF:**

2 pounds lean ground beef

¾ cup quick oats

1 egg

⅔ cup tomato juice

1 small onion, chopped

½ teaspoon pepper

1 teaspoon salt

**SAUCE:**

⅓ cup ketchup

1 tablespoon Dijon mustard

1 tablespoon brown sugar

1. Preheat oven to 350°F.
2. Mix all the meat loaf ingredients together in a large bowl; shape into a loaf. Place into a 9" × 5" × 3" pan.
3. Mix sauce ingredients together and set aside.
4. Bake the meat loaf for 45 minutes. Remove from oven and pour sauce evenly over the top. Return the meat loaf to the oven and continue to cook for another 30 minutes.

SERVES 8

**THE F-FACTOR DIET NUTRITIONAL CONTENT FOR JOURNALING**
Per Serving: 7 g carbohydrate • 1 g fiber

**ACTUAL NUTRITIONAL CONTENT**
Per Serving: 319 calories • 11 g carbohydrate • 1 g fiber • 23 g protein • 20 g total fat • 8 g sat. fat • 581 mg sodium

# Zucchini Noodle Bolognese

STEPS 2 AND 3

*Spaghetti Bolognese is my absolute favorite food, but a big bowl of cooked spaghetti can be over 400 calories—before the sauce! A medium zucchini is only about 33 calories to begin with, meaning I can have more and more, without the guilt.*

> 3 large zucchini
> 2 tablespoons olive oil
> 1 large onion, diced
> 2 stalks celery, diced
> 2 large carrots, diced (should yield 1 cup)
> 1 1-pound package lean ground beef
> 7 cloves garlic, diced
> 1 cup dry red wine
> 1 28-ounce can crushed tomatoes
> 2 tablespoons tomato paste
> 1 cup whole milk
> 2-inch rind from Parmesan cheese
> 1 teaspoon oregano
> salt and pepper to taste
> ¼ cup grated Parmesan cheese

1. Wash and spiralize zucchini using a spiralizer, mandoline, or peeler to form noodles or ribbons. Set aside on paper towels so that any excess water is soaked up. Feel free to sprinkle with a pinch of kosher salt to help with this.
2. Add 1 tablespoon olive oil to a large saucepan over medium heat and sauté diced onion, celery, and carrots until soft, about 5 minutes.
3. Add ground beef and cook until crumbled and brown, draining excess liquid as necessary.
4. Add garlic and sauté for another minute.
5. Add dry red wine and scrape the bottom of the pan. Bring the wine to a boil and cook for another 5 minutes until the wine has cooked off and the pan is dry.
6. Add crushed tomatoes, tomato paste, whole milk, Parmesan cheese rind, dried oregano, salt, and pepper to the skillet. Stir well and bring to a boil.
7. Once mixture is boiling, reduce heat and simmer for an additional 10 to 15 minutes.

8. While sauce is cooking, sauté zucchini noodles in another pan with 1 tablespoon olive oil over medium-high heat for 1 to 2 minutes, until tender. Remove from heat and season with salt and pepper as desired.

9. After sauce has cooked for 10 to 15 minutes, remove Parmesan rind and remove from heat. Stir in ¼ cup grated Parmesan.

10. Top zoodles with the Bolognese sauce, serve, and enjoy!

SERVES 6

**THE F-FACTOR DIET NUTRITIONAL CONTENT FOR JOURNALING**
Per Serving: 4 g carbohydrate • 6 g fiber

**ACTUAL NUTRITIONAL CONTENT**
Per Serving: 310 calories • 27 g carbohydrate • 6 g fiber • 25 g protein • 10 g fat • 3 g sat. fat • 425 mg sodium

✳ FISH AND SHELLFISH MAIN DISHES

# Crispy Oven-Fried Fish

STEPS 2 AND 3

*Growing up, the only fish I would eat was Arthur Treacher's fried fish n' chips. The thick coating of fried batter completely overpowered the fish—which is probably why I liked it so much. Here is a grown-up, much healthier version. Pair it with sweet potato chips (p. 233) for a true fish and chips meal!*

1 pound fresh fish fillets, ½ inch thick (orange roughy, skinless cod, or catfish fillets)
¼ cup skim milk
½ cup whole-wheat flour
⅓ cup seasoned bread crumbs
¼ cup grated Parmesan cheese
⅛ teaspoon pepper
nonstick cooking spray

1. Preheat oven to 450°F.
2. Rinse fish; pat dry with paper towels.

3. Place milk in a shallow dish.
4. In another shallow dish, combine flour, bread crumbs, Parmesan cheese, and pepper.
5. Dip each piece of fish in the milk, then in the bread crumb mixture. Coat both sides and place on a baking sheet coated with nonstick spray.
6. Spray tops of fillets with nonstick spray and bake for 7 to 9 minutes, or until fish flakes easily with a fork.

SERVES 4

**THE F-FACTOR DIET NUTRITIONAL CONTENT FOR JOURNALING**
Per Serving: 19 g carbohydrate • 2 g fiber

**ACTUAL NUTRITIONAL CONTENT**
Per Serving: 213 calories • 19 g carbohydrate • 2 g fiber • 27 g protein • 3 g total fat • 1 g sat. fat • 357 mg sodium

# Tuna and White Bean Salad

STEPS 2 AND 3

*This is a great salad to make on summer days when you don't want to be stuck in the kitchen for hours slaving over a hot stove. This salad couldn't be easier to prepare and takes just a few minutes to toss the ingredients together. It is popular in Italy, and the combination of high-fiber beans and lean protein in the tuna makes it an ideal meal to enjoy on the F-Factor Diet.*

2 cups string beans, washed and ends trimmed
1 7-ounce can water-packed tuna, drained
¾ cup red onion, thinly sliced
½ cup celery, thinly chopped
1 15.5-ounce can white beans (cannellini), drained and rinsed
1 tablespoon olive oil
1 tablespoon red wine vinegar
1 tablespoon chopped Italian parsley
8 cups arugula

1. Fill a large pot with water and bring to a boil. Add string beans and cook for 3 minutes, until al dente. Drain the string beans and place in a bowl of ice water to prevent further cooking. When fully cooled, remove string beans, dry, and cut into bite-sized pieces.
2. Place the tuna in a large bowl and break up with a fork.
3. Stir in onion, celery, white beans, string beans, salt, and pepper.
4. Add oil, vinegar, and parsley and toss gently to combine.
5. Place arugula on a large serving platter and top with tuna salad.

SERVES 4

**THE F-FACTOR DIET NUTRITIONAL CONTENT FOR JOURNALING**
Per Serving: 15 g carbohydrate • 7 g fiber

**ACTUAL NUTRITIONAL CONTENT**
Per Serving: 243 calories • 28 g carbohydrate • 7 g fiber • 22 g protein • 5 g total fat • 1 g sat. fat • 433 mg sodium

## Broiled Snapper with Black Bean Salsa

STEPS 2 AND 3

*This dish is reminiscent of one I had in Cabo San Lucas, Mexico. The Mexican flavors will wake up your palate. The avocado adds a good source of monoun-saturated fat. This dish has it all: heart-healthy fat, a good serving of fiber, plus lean protein. You will feel full and satisfied long after your plate is clean.*

1 15.5-ounce can black beans, rinsed and drained

2 navel oranges, peeled and chopped

1 medium tomato, seeded and chopped

½ cup plus 2 tablespoons fresh cilantro, chopped

1 jalapeño pepper, seeded and minced finely

2½ tablespoons fresh lime juice

salt and pepper

1 avocado, peeled and chopped

4 red snapper fillets, 5 ounces each

2 tablespoons olive oil

1. Combine black beans, oranges, tomato, ½ cup cilantro, jalapeño pepper, and lime juice ingredients in a medium bowl.
2. Season the salsa with salt and pepper to taste. Mix avocado into the salsa and refrigerate until ready to serve.
3. Brush fish with oil and sprinkle with salt and pepper. Broil or grill until just cooked through (about 9 minutes per inch of thickness if broiling). Transfer fish to plates and sprinkle with chopped fresh cilantro. Serve fish with salsa.

SERVES 4

**THE F-FACTOR DIET NUTRITIONAL CONTENT FOR JOURNALING**
Per Serving: 43 g carbohydrate • 12 g fiber

**ACTUAL NUTRITIONAL CONTENT**
Per Serving: 483 calories • 43 g carbohydrate • 12 g fiber • 42 g protein • 17 g total fat • 3 g sat. fat • 102 mg sodium

## Zesty Shrimp Burritos

STEPS 2 AND 3

*These high-fiber burritos will satisfy even the most devoted Mexican-food lover. They have great flavor and texture, minus the fat of a meat version. Serve with a green salad. (Note: Many fish counters will clean shrimp for you at little or no cost.)*

1 pound fresh shrimp, cleaned, shelled, and deveined
nonstick cooking spray
1 small onion, chopped
½ green pepper, chopped
½ red pepper, chopped
1 cup frozen corn kernels, defrosted
2 tablespoons green chili peppers, chopped
1 clove garlic, minced
¼ cup water
1 tablespoon chili powder

1 tablespoon ground cumin
⅛ teaspoon salt
1 cup cooked brown rice
8 La Tortilla Factory whole-wheat low-carb/low-fat tortillas
1½ cups reduced-fat shredded cheddar cheese
2 cups spinach leaves, steamed

1. Chop shrimp into bite-sized pieces.
2. Heat a large skillet and spray with nonstick spray. Sauté onion, green and red peppers, corn, green chili pepper, and garlic until the vegetables are tender (about 3 minutes). Add the shrimp, water, chili powder, cumin, and salt and cook about 5 minutes or until most of the water has evaporated. Remove from heat and stir in brown rice.
3. Meanwhile, place tortillas between two damp paper towels and microwave on high for 20 seconds to soften for easier rolling, or warm in a 200°F oven.
4. Spoon ½ cup of shrimp filling onto the center of each tortilla. Top with 2 tablespoons of cheese and ¼ cup spinach. Fold bottom edge of each tortilla up and over filling. Fold the opposite sides in, just until they meet. Roll up from the bottom.
5. Arrange burritos on a baking sheet, seam sides down. Bake in a 350°F oven for 10 minutes until heated through.
6. Serve warm.

SERVES 8

**THE F-FACTOR DIET NUTRITIONAL CONTENT FOR JOURNALING**
Per Burrito: 32 g carbohydrate • 16 g fiber

**ACTUAL NUTRITIONAL CONTENT**
Per Serving: 237 calories • 32 g carbohydrate • 16 g fiber • 27 g protein • 6 g total fat • 1 g sat. fat • 546 mg sodium

# Thai Shrimp Summer Rolls

STEPS 2 AND 3

*This refreshing summer appetizer is one of my favorites—not only does it look pretty, but it tastes great, too!*

2 ounces (⅓ package prepared) **Miracle Noodle Angel Hair Shirataki Pasta**

12 rounds rice paper

24 large peeled and cooked shrimp

1 large avocado, cut into strips

2 cups shredded carrot

3 cups shredded red cabbage

¼ cup cilantro

1 cup basil, chopped

1 cup mint leaves, chopped

DIPPING SAUCE INGREDIENTS:

¼ cup PB2 powdered peanut butter

1 tablespoon reduced-sodium soy sauce

2 teaspoons sriracha

1 teaspoon grated ginger

¼ cup warm water

1. Prepare Miracle Noodles according to directions on package. Cut prepared noodles into 3-inch pieces and set aside.
2. Prepare dipping sauce by mixing together dipping sauce ingredients. Set aside.
3. Lay out remaining ingredients. Take a rice paper wrapper and completely submerge it in hot water 10 to 15 seconds, until pliable.
4. Place the wrapper on a plate and fill with prepared Miracle Noodles, 2 shrimp, a slice of avocado, carrots, cabbage, cilantro, basil, and mint. Fold the bottom half of the wrapper over the filling, hold the fold in place, tuck in the sides, and roll tightly.

5. Repeat with remaining rice paper wrappers and fillings and serve with dipping sauce.

SERVES 12

**THE F-FACTOR DIET NUTRITIONAL CONTENT FOR JOURNALING**
Per Serving: 11 g carbohydrate • 2 g fiber

**ACTUAL NUTRITIONAL CONTENT**
Per Serving: 96 calories • 15 g carbohydrate • 2 g fiber • 5 g protein • 2 g fat • 0 g sat. fat • 135 mg sodium

✳ PASTA AND GRAINS

# Pasta Bolognese

STEPS 2 AND 3

*I love a good Bolognese sauce, yet every time I made it at home, it always seemed to be missing an ingredient that I tasted in Italian restaurants. One day, while watching Mario Batali on the Food Network, I found out what it was—milk! The addition of milk makes this sauce creamy and luxurious and gives it the light pink hue I was accustomed to seeing in the restaurants. Mystery solved!*

2 tablespoons olive oil
1 small onion, finely chopped
2 celery ribs, finally chopped
2 carrots, finely chopped
2 garlic cloves, minced
1 pound extra-lean ground beef
½ pound ground pork
½ pound ground turkey breast
1 cup dry red wine
2 cups skim milk
1 cup crushed tomatoes
1 cup beef broth
2 tablespoons tomato paste

1 teaspoon oregano
½ teaspoon salt
¼ teaspoon pepper
1 pound whole-wheat blend spaghetti

1. Heat the oil in a large Dutch oven over medium-high heat.
2. Stir in the onion, celery, carrot, and garlic, and cook until the celery and onion are soft, about 5 minutes.
3. Add the ground beef, ground pork, and ground turkey breast, stirring and breaking the meat up. Cook until the meat is no longer pink.
4. Add the wine, and cook until the liquid has evaporated.
5. Add the milk, crushed red tomatoes, beef broth, tomato paste, and seasonings. Reduce heat and simmer for 1 hour.
6. In a large pot of salted boiling water, cook pasta according to package directions or until desired consistency.
7. Drain pasta, place in a large bowl, and top with Bolognese sauce.

SERVES 8

**THE F-FACTOR DIET NUTRITIONAL CONTENT FOR JOURNALING**
Per Serving: 53 g carbohydrate • 8 g fiber

**ACTUAL NUTRITIONAL CONTENT**
Per Serving: 420 calories • 53 g carbohydrate • 8 g fiber • 26 g protein • 20 g total fat • 7 g sat. fat • 375 mg sodium

# Macaroni and Cheese

STEPS 2 AND 3

*Good old mac and cheese is perhaps the ultimate comfort food, but it usually comes with the burden of more than 20 grams of fat per serving. I eliminated the guilt—but not the flavor—by using low-fat milk, reduced-fat cheese, and a fiber-rich pasta.*

1 cup 1% low-fat milk
1 cup 1% low-fat cottage cheese

1½ cups shredded reduced-fat cheddar cheese

¼ teaspoon salt

⅛ teaspoon pepper

1 pound Barilla Plus multigrain elbow pasta

3 tablespoons bread crumbs

1. Preheat oven to 400°F. Bring a large pot of water to a boil for the pasta.
2. In a saucepan, bring the milk to a boil. Lower the heat and stir in the cottage cheese, cheddar cheese, salt, and pepper. Stir until the cheese is melted and keep warm.
3. Cook pasta until tender but firm. Drain pasta and return to its pot. Add the cheese sauce to the pasta and stir well to combine. Transfer the mixture to a baking or casserole dish and sprinkle the top with bread crumbs.
4. Bake for 25 to 30 minutes until bubbly and the top is golden. Serve immediately.

SERVES 4

**THE F-FACTOR DIET NUTRITIONAL CONTENT FOR JOURNALING**
Per Serving: 40 g carbohydrate • 5 g fiber

**ACTUAL NUTRITIONAL CONTENT**
Per Serving: 410 calories • 40 g carbohydrate • 5 g fiber • 26 g protein • 5 g total fat • 3 g sat. fat • 715 mg sodium

## Linguine with Clam Sauce

STEPS 2 AND 3

*Clams provide a good source of protein, vitamins, and minerals including omega-3 fatty acids and iron. Clams are also low in calories, fat, and cholesterol. This is a pasta sauce you can feel good about eating!*

8 ounces Barilla White Fiber Thin Spaghetti

2 tablespoons olive oil

2 garlic cloves, minced

2 tablespoons diced shallots

⅓ cup dry white wine

¼ teaspoon black pepper

1 26-ounce jar tomato sauce

1 14-ounce jar artichoke hearts, drained and quartered

1 10-ounce can baby clams, undrained

2 tablespoons chopped fresh basil, or 2 teaspoons dried basil

2 tablespoons chopped fresh parsley

1. Bring a large pot of water to a boil. Add pasta and cook for 8 to 10 minutes.
2. Meanwhile, heat the oil in a large saucepan over medium-high heat. Add the garlic and shallots, and sauté 2 minutes or until tender. Add the wine and the next 4 ingredients (pepper through clams). Reduce heat, and simmer for 5 minutes. Stir in basil and parsley.
3. Drain pasta and place in a serving bowl. Serve sauce over pasta.

SERVES 4

**THE F-FACTOR DIET NUTRITIONAL CONTENT FOR JOURNALING**
Per Serving: 45 g carbohydrate • 10 g fiber

**ACTUAL NUTRITIONAL CONTENT**
Per Serving: 285 calories • 47 g carbohydrate • 7 g fiber • 8 g protein • 7 g total fat • 1 g sat. fat • 1275 mg sodium

## Nutty Stir-Fried Rice

STEPS 2 AND 3

*The fried rice served in Chinese restaurants is usually made with white rice and a ton of oil—tasty, but a nightmare if you're watching your weight. Typical fried rice can have as much as 400 calories and 15 grams of fat per cup. Reducing the oil, substituting brown rice for white, and adding good fiber-rich vegetables not only lowers the fat and calories but results in a dish that is healthy and filling.*

1 teaspoon vegetable oil

1 clove garlic, minced

1 cup broccoli florets, chopped

1 cup red bell pepper, seeded and diced
1 carrot, peeled and diced
1 onion, chopped
½ cup mushrooms, sliced thin
4 ounces cooked chicken breast, chopped
3 cups cooked brown rice
2 tablespoons chopped peanuts
2 tablespoons low-sodium soy sauce

1. Heat the oil in a large nonstick skillet or a wok over high heat.
2. Sauté the garlic until golden brown, then add the broccoli, pepper, carrots, and onion. Sauté until crisp and tender, then add the mushrooms. Cook briefly until all the vegetables are crisp and tender.
3. Add the chicken, rice, peanuts, and soy sauce. Stir-fry for another minute until all the ingredients are mixed and cooked through.

SERVES 4

**THE F-FACTOR DIET NUTRITIONAL CONTENT FOR JOURNALING**
Per Serving: 34 g carbohydrate • 5 g fiber

**ACTUAL NUTRITIONAL CONTENT**
Per Serving: 287 calories • 44 g carbohydrate • 4 g fiber • 15 g protein • 6 g total fat • 1 g sat. fat • 844 mg sodium

## Quinoa and Chickpea Burgers in Lettuce Wraps

STEPS 2 AND 3

*These quinoa and chickpea burgers are full of protein, fiber, and flavor! I can taste the yumminess already.*

½ cup white quinoa
1 cup low-sodium vegetable broth
2 small slices whole-wheat bread
1 14-ounce can chickpeas, drained and rinsed
1 large egg

¼ cup cilantro leaves
1 teaspoon cumin
1 small red chili
salt and black pepper
1 tablespoon vegetable oil
2 heads butter lettuce, washed, core removed

1. In a saucepan, bring quinoa and broth to a boil over medium-high heat.
2. Cover, reduce heat to low, and cook until all broth has been absorbed, about 15 minutes. Let cool slightly.
3. In a food processor, process bread until fine bread crumbs form. Add chickpeas, quinoa, egg, cilantro, cumin, chili, salt, and pepper and process in short bursts until mixture is finely chopped.
4. Shape mixture into 4 patties. Brush patties with oil and cook in a nonstick frying pan over medium-high heat until golden, about 4 minutes per side.
5. Place the patties on the lettuce leaves and enjoy.

SERVES 4

**THE F-FACTOR DIET NUTRITIONAL CONTENT FOR JOURNALING**
Per Serving: 24 g carbohydrate • 7 g fiber

**ACTUAL NUTRITIONAL CONTENT**
Per Serving: 212 calories • 27 g carbohydrate • 7 g fiber • 11 g protein • 8 g fat • 4 g sat. fat • 1006 mg sodium

# Tabouli Salad

STEPS 2 AND 3

*Tabouli salad is a staple of the Mediterranean diet. This salad is delicious alongside shrimp with feta cheese.*

½ cup bulgur
3 plum tomatoes, seeded and finely chopped
1 green pepper, seeded and finely chopped
1 medium onion, finely chopped

1 cucumber, seeded and finely chopped

1 cup fresh parsley, chopped

1 tablespoon chopped fresh mint

½ cup lemon juice

¼ teaspoon salt

2 tablespoons olive oil

1. Place bulgur in a glass bowl and cover with boiling water. Let sit for about 15 to 20 minutes. Drain well.
2. Add the tomatoes, green pepper, onion, cucumber, parsley, and mint.
3. In a small bowl, whisk together the lemon juice, salt, and olive oil. Pour over bulgur and toss well to coat evenly.
4. Serve.

SERVES 4

**THE F-FACTOR DIET NUTRITIONAL CONTENT FOR JOURNALING**
Per Serving: 20 g carbohydrate • 6 g fiber

**ACTUAL NUTRITIONAL CONTENT**
Per Serving: 171 calories • 26 g carbohydrate • 6 g fiber • 4 g protein • 7 g total fat • 1 g sat. fat • 165 mg sodium

✳ SWEETS

# Chocolate-Cherry-Almond Biscotti

STEPS 2 AND 3

*Whenever I bake these, they're eaten up in a flash. No one can resist these cookies, and the best part is, no one realizes that they are low in fat and calories, and even deliver a gram of fiber.*

1 cup white flour

1 cup whole-wheat flour

½ cup unsweetened cocoa powder

1 teaspoon baking powder

¼ teaspoon salt

1 whole egg

2 egg whites

1 cup Truvia

1 tablespoon almond extract

1 cup dried cherries

1 cup slivered almonds

1. Preheat oven to 350°F.
2. Sift together flours, cocoa powder, baking powder, and salt.
3. In a large bowl, beat egg, egg whites, and sweetener with a mixer until thick. Add almond extract, cherries, and almonds. Mix for 10 seconds.
4. Add dry ingredients to wet and combine until mixture is moistened. The dough will be very sticky.
5. Flour a board and turn dough out onto it. Divide dough in half.
6. Roll each half into a 13" × 2" log. Place on a nonstick cookie sheet and bake for 30 minutes or until dough is golden and cracked on top.
7. Remove from oven and let cool 10 minutes. Lower oven temperature to 325°F. Cut each log on the bias in ¼-inch slices (use a serrated knife for easier slicing). Place the slices flat in the pan and bake 4 to 5 minutes on each side.
8. Let cool (they get harder once they are cooled off completely) and serve.

MAKES 50 COOKIES

**THE F-FACTOR DIET NUTRITIONAL CONTENT FOR JOURNALING**
Per Cookie: 11 g carbohydrate • 1 g fiber

**ACTUAL NUTRITIONAL CONTENT**
Per Serving: 62 calories • 11 g carbohydrate • 1 g fiber • 2 g protein • 2 g total fat • 0 g sat. fat • 26 mg sodium

# Cinnamon Sugar Skinny Chips

STEPS 2 AND 3

*My communications director, Jessica, is always saying how cinnamon sugar pita chips are her weakness. This recipe is the solution to the sweet-savory chip conundrum.*

> nonstick cooking spray
> 1 tablespoon F-Factor Vanilla Fiber/Protein Powder
> 2 tablespoons Truvia
> 1 tablespoon cinnamon
> 6 6-inch corn tortillas

1. Preheat oven to 350°F. Coat a baking sheet with nonstick cooking spray.
2. In a bowl, mix protein powder, Truvia, and cinnamon.
3. Take each corn tortilla and coat each side with nonstick cooking spray. Sprinkle with dry mixture and place on prepared baking sheet.
4. Using a knife or pizza cutter, cut each tortilla into 8 triangle shapes (i.e., chips).
5. Place on a baking sheet, sprinkle remaining vanilla-cinnamon-sugar mixture on top, and pop in oven for 12 to 15 minutes, or until edges begin to brown.
6. Remove from oven and allow to cool.

SERVES 3 (16 CHIPS PER SERVING)

**THE F-FACTOR DIET NUTRITIONAL CONTENT FOR JOURNALING**
Per Serving: 25 g carbohydrate • 6 g fiber

**ACTUAL NUTRITIONAL CONTENT**
Per Serving: 120 calories • 25 g carbohydrate • 6 g fiber • 5 g protein • 2 g fat • 0 g sat. fat • 29 mg sodium

# Cranberry-Walnut Chutney

STEPS 2 AND 3

*This recipe won best "surprise" dish at a potluck luncheon contest my mom attended. It wasn't her entry, but she did manage to get the recipe. It's delicious on its own, as a side dish for roasted meat, or even as a dessert topping.*

4 cups fresh cranberries
2 cups Truvia
½ cup walnuts (roasted)
4 ounces low-sugar orange marmalade

1. Mix together all the ingredients and place in a 7" × 12" ovenproof dish. Bake at 350°F for ½ hour.
2. Chill.

SERVES 8

**THE F-FACTOR DIET NUTRITIONAL CONTENT FOR JOURNALING**
Per Serving: 13 g carbohydrate • 3 g fiber

**ACTUAL NUTRITIONAL CONTENT**
Per Serving: 90 calories • 13 g carbohydrate • 3 g fiber • 1 g protein • 4 g total fat • 0 g sat. fat • 1 mg sodium

# Berry Crisp

STEPS 2 AND 3

*This is my favorite dessert in the book. I love warm cobblers and crisps, and this one fits the bill. It tastes decadent, but is surprisingly low in calories and fat. Serving with a dollop of So Delicious CocoWhip! makes this a truly special treat.*

FRUIT:
4 cups mixed frozen berries (blueberries, raspberries, blackberries), thawed
½ teaspoon cinnamon
2 teaspoons Truvia

TOPPING:

1 cup almond meal/flour

1 cup quick-cooking rolled oats

2 tablespoons Truvia, or other non-nutritive sweetener

½ cup softened butter

½ teaspoon cinnamon

½ teaspoon nutmeg

1 teaspoon vanilla

½ cup chopped walnuts (optional)

1. Preheat oven to 350°F.
2. Place berries in bottom of pie plate and sprinkle with cinnamon and Truvia. Toss to coat and set aside.
3. In a medium bowl, place almond meal, oats, sweetener, butter, cinnamon, nutmeg and vanilla. Cut together with fork until a dough is formed. Stir in walnuts until well incorporated.
4. Using your fingers, pinch off bits of topping and place all over top of berries. Bake at 350°F for 30 minutes or until lightly browned.

SERVES 10

**THE F-FACTOR DIET NUTRITIONAL CONTENT FOR JOURNALING (WITH WALNUTS)**
Per Serving: 17 g carbohydrate • 4 g fiber

**ACTUAL NUTRITIONAL CONTENT (WITH WALNUTS)**
Per Serving: 222 calories • 17 g carbohydrate • 4 g fiber • 6 g protein • 16 g total fat • 6 g sat. fat • 147 mg sodium

## Chocolate-Covered Bananas

STEPS 2 AND 3

*These are great plain, but you can get creative with optional coatings. Chocolate sprinkles, chopped nuts, and shredded coconut are all delicious!*

3 ripe bananas

7 ounces semisweet chocolate chips

1. Peel bananas and cut in half crosswise. Insert a wooden stick into the flat end of each banana half. Lay bananas on a shallow pan and freeze for about 3 hours.
2. Place chocolate chips in a microwave-safe bowl. Place in microwave and cook on high for 40 seconds. Stir until smooth.
3. With a spatula, spread chocolate over each banana. The chocolate will harden immediately. Wrap each banana in plastic wrap and place in the freezer until you are ready to eat them. Yes—straight from the freezer!

SERVES 6

**THE F-FACTOR DIET NUTRITIONAL CONTENT FOR JOURNALING**
Per Serving: 35 g carbohydrate • 3 g fiber

**ACTUAL NUTRITIONAL CONTENT**
Per Serving: 213 calories • 35 g carbohydrate • 3 g fiber • 2 g protein • 10 g total fat • 6 g sat. fat • 4 mg sodium

# FIBER CONTENT OF POPULAR FOODS

## Carbohydrate and Fiber Content of Common Foods Not on the Exchange Lists

### *(See pages 31–42 for the Exchange Lists)*

|  | *Carb grams* | *Fiber grams* |
|---|---|---|
| **BREADS** | | |
| challah, 1 slice | 15 | 1 |
| sprouted grain bread, 1 slice | 15 | 2 |
| **CRACKERS** | | |
| flax seed crackers (Flackers), 8 crackers | 7 | 6 |
| **MISCELLANEOUS** | | |
| chia seeds, 1 tbsp. | 6 | 5 |
| flax seeds, 1 tbsp. | 3 | 3 |
| hemp seeds, 3 tbsp. | 3 | 1 |
| PB2 powdered peanut butter, 2 tbsp. | 5 | 2 |

|  | Carb grams | Fiber grams |
|---|---|---|
| **FRUITS** | | |
| guava, 1 fruit | 8 | 3 |
| lychee, ½ cup | 15 | 1 |
| passion fruit, ¼ cup | 15 | 6 |
| **GRAINS** | | |
| buckwheat, ⅛ cup | 15 | 2 |
| farro, ⅓ cup | 40 | 4 |
| quinoa, ⅓ cup cooked | 15 | 3 |
| rice noodles, ⅓ cup | 15 | 1 |
| spelt, ⅓ cup | 15 | 3 |
| **NONSTARCHY VEGETABLES (1 CUP RAW, ½ CUP COOKED)** | | |
| baby corn | 0 | 2 |
| bok choy | 0 | 2 |
| hearts of palm | 0 | 4 |
| jicama | 0 | 6 |
| pickles | 0 | 1 |
| sauerkraut | 0 | 4 |
| seaweed | 0 | 1 |
| shishito peppers | 0 | 2 |
| sugar snap peas | 0 | 3 |
| **STARCHY VEGETABLES AND LEGUMES** | | |
| barley, ⅓ cup | 15 | 2 |
| spaghetti squash, 1 cup cooked | 15 | 3 |
| taro, ½ cup | 15 | 2 |
| **BEVERAGES** | | |
| bouillon or broth, 8 fl. oz | 1 | 0 |
| club soda or mineral water, 8 fl. oz | 0 | 0 |
| coffee or tea, 6 fl. oz | 0 | 0 |
| cranberry juice cocktail, 8 fl. oz | 33–36 | 0 |
| fruit drinks & sweet teas, 8 fl. oz | 25–35 | 0 |
| soft drinks, 12 fl. oz | 32–46 | 0 |

|  | Carb grams | Fiber grams |
|---|---|---|
| diet soft drinks, 12 fl. oz | 0 | 0 |
| sports drinks, 12 fl. oz | 21–30 | 0 |
| beer, regular, 12 fl. oz | 13 | 0 |
| light beer, 12 fl. oz | 4–5 | 0 |
| nonalcoholic beer, 12 fl. oz | 10–20 | 0 |
| daiquiri or margarita, 7 fl. oz | 33 | 0 |
| gin, rum, vodka, whiskey, 1 fl. oz | 0 | 0 |
| liqueur, coffee flavored, 1.5 fl. oz | 24 | 0 |
| tonic water/collins mixer, 8 fl. oz | 22 | 0 |
| wine, red or white, 4 fl. oz | 2 | 0 |
| wine, sweet dessert, 2 fl. oz | 7 | 0 |

## SNACKS & DESSERTS

|  | Carb grams | Fiber grams |
|---|---|---|
| beef jerky, 1 large piece, 1 oz | 2–3 | 1 |
| **CAKE,** 1/12 of 9" cake, no frosting | | |
| angel food, from mix | 29 | 0 |
| chocolate, from recipe | 51 | 2 |
| white, from recipe | 42 | 1 |
| frosting, ½ cup or recipe | 26 | 0 |
| candy bar, 1.75–2 oz | 30 | 2 |
| **CHIPS:** potato, 1 oz, about 20 | 15 | 1 |
| tortilla chips, 1 oz, 8–12 | 18 | 2 |
| **COOKIES, BARS, & SNACK CAKES:** | | |
| brownie, from mix, 2" square | 25 | 0 |
| packaged cookie, 1 | 10 | 0 |
| graham crackers, 1 sheet | 11 | 0 |
| granola or cereal bar, 1 oz | 20 | 1 |
| snack cake, 1 cupcake | 30 | 0 |
| **FROZEN & CHILLED SNACKS:** | | |
| frozen yogurt | 40 | >1 |
| fruit or juice bar, 1 | 6–23 | 0 |
| gelatin dessert, 1 cup | 38 | 0 |
| sugar-free gelatin, 1 cup | 0 | 0 |

| | Carb grams | Fiber grams |
|---|---|---|
| ice cream, 1 cup | 30–40 | 0 |
| sugar-free ice cream, 1 cup | 22–40 | 0 |
| nondairy frozen dessert | 20–50 | 0 |
| sherbet or sorbet, 1 cup | 50–60 | 0 |
| frozen burrito, beef & bean, 5 oz | 40–50 | 5 |
| frozen pizza, 7" single | 25–50 | 2 |
| **PIE,** ⅙ of 9" pie, from recipe | | |
| apple | 77 | 2 |
| lemon meringue | 67 | 1 |
| pecan | 85 | 4 |
| pumpkin | 55 | 3 |
| **POPCORN,** 5 cups popped | 25 | 5 |
| caramel corn with peanuts, 1 cup | 35 | 2 |
| popcorn cake or rice cake, 1 | 7 | 0 |
| pork skins, 1 ounce | 0 | 0 |
| pretzels, 1 ounce | 22 | 0 |
| **PUDDING,** ½ cup | 20–30 | 0 |
| sugar-free pudding, ½ cup | 12 | 0 |
| pumpkin seeds, ¼ cup kernels | 8 | 2 |
| sunflower seeds, ¼ cup kernels | 8 | 3 |
| trail mix, ¼ cup | 16–23 | 3 |

## BAKING INGREDIENTS

| | | |
|---|---|---|
| biscuit mix, 1 cup | 75 | 0 |
| brown sugar, 1 cup, packed | 214 | 0 |
| chocolate chips, 1 cup | 110 | 0 |
| coconut, 1 cup | 44 | 8 |
| corn syrup, 1 cup | 250 | 0 |
| flour, all-purpose, 1 cup | 85 | 0 |
| marshmallows, 1 cup | 46 | 0 |
| oatmeal, 1 cup | 57 | 9 |
| oil or shortening, 1 cup | 0 | 0 |
| powdered sugar, 1 cup | 120 | 0 |
| white granulated sugar, 1 cup | 200 | 0 |

## FAST FOODS

Ask for nutritional information where you buy fast food.

| | *Carb grams* | *Fiber grams* |
|---|---|---|
| **JAMBA JUICE:** 24-oz smoothie | 57–110 | 2–6 |
| **KFC:** original recipe breast | 11 | 2 |
| extra crispy breast | 18 | 0 |
| thigh, any variety | 0–10 | 0–1 |
| chicken pot pie | 66 | 3 |
| mashed potatoes w/gravy | 19 | 1 |
| **McDONALD'S:** Big Mac® | 46 | 3 |
| hamburger or cheeseburger | 31–33 | 2 |
| Filet-o-Fish® | 39 | 2 |
| French fries, medium | 44 | 4 |
| Bacon Ranch Grilled Chicken Salad | 9 | 3 |
| Egg McMuffin® | 30 | 2 |
| hotcakes with syrup | 102 | 2 |
| fruit 'n yogurt parfait, 5.3 oz | 30 | 1 |
| McFlurry®, Oreo, regular size | 60 | 1 |
| **PANDA EXPRESS:** egg roll, 1 | 20 | 2 |
| beef and broccoli, 5.5 oz | 13 | 2 |
| orange chicken, 5.7 oz | 44 | 0 |
| vegetable chow mein, 9.4 oz | 80 | 6 |
| **PIZZA HUT:** most varieties | | |
| hand tossed, 1 slice | 26 | 2 |
| personal pan, 1 pizza | 69 | 6 |
| **SUBWAY:** most 6" sandwiches | 41–58 | 2–6 |
| breakfast sandwiches | 43–45 | 2 |
| **TACO BELL:** taco | 13 | 3 |
| soft taco, chicken | 16 | 1 |
| Supreme Beef Burrito | 51 | 8 |
| Nachos Supreme | 46 | 8 |
| Nachos BellGrande | 84 | 13 |

|  | Carb grams | Fiber grams |
| --- | --- | --- |
| taco salad with shell | 77 | 11 |
| Power Menu Bowl, Chicken | 53 | 8 |
| Chalupa Supreme chicken | 31 | 2 |
| **WENDY'S:** chili, 12 oz | 23 | 5 |
| classic single w/everything | 39 | 3 |
| spicy chicken sandwich | 51 | 3 |
| Power Mediterranean Chicken Salad | 42 | 8 |
| baked potato, broccoli & cheese | 70 | 10 |
| frosty, 16 oz | 76 | 0 |

## RECOMMENDED CEREALS AND BREADS

## Cereals

### All-Bran Bran Buds
Serving Size: ⅓ cup
Calories: 80
Total Carbohydrate: 24 g
Fiber: 13 g
Net Carbohydrate: 11 g

### All-Bran Complete Wheat Flakes
Serving Size: ¾ cup
Calories: 90
Total Carbohydrate: 23 g
Fiber: 5 g
Net Carbohydrate: 19 g

### All-Bran Original
Serving Size: ⅓ cup
Calories: 80
Total Carbohydrate: 23 g
Fiber: 10 g
Net Carbohydrate: 13 g

### Barbara's Bakery Puffins Cinnamon Flavor
Serving Size: ⅔ cup
Calories: 90
Total Carbohydrate: 24 g
Fiber: 5 g
Net Carbohydrate: 19 g

**Barbara's Bakery Puffins Original**
Serving Size: ¾ cup
Calories: 90
Total Carbohydrate: 24 g
Fiber: 5 g
Net Carbohydrate: 19 g

**Fiber One**
Serving Size: ½ cup
Calories: 60
Total Carbohydrate: 25 g
Fiber: 14 g
Net Carbohydrate: 11 g

**Fiber One Honey Clusters**
Serving Size: 1 cup
Calories: 170
Total Carbohydrate: 44 g
Fiber: 10 g
Net Carbohydrate: 34 g

**General Mills Wheat Chex**
Serving Size: ¾ cup
Calories: 160
Total Carbohydrate: 39 g
Fiber: 6 g
Net Carbohydrate: 33 g

**Kashi Go Lean**
Serving Size: 1¼ cup
Calories: 180
Total Carbohydrate: 40 g
Fiber: 13 g
Net Carbohydrate: 27 g

**Kashi Go Lean Crisp! Cinnamon Crumble**
Serving Size: ¾ cup
Calories: 180
Total Carbohydrate: 32 g
Fiber: 9 g
Net Carbohydrate: 23 g

**Nature's Path Organic Optimum Power Blueberry Cinnamon Flax Cereal**
Serving Size: ¾ cup
Calories: 200
Total Carbohydrate: 38 g
Fiber: 9 g
Net Carbohydrate: 29 g

**Nature's Path SmartBran**
Serving Size: ½ cup
Calories: 80
Total Carbohydrate: 24 g
Fiber: 13 g
Net Carbohydrate: 11 g

**Nutritious Living Hi-Lo**
Serving Size: ½ cup
Calories: 90
Total Carbohydrate: 13 g
Fiber: 7 g
Net Carbohydrate: 6 g

**Quaker Instant Oatmeal Weight Control**
Serving Size: 1 packet
Calories: 160

Total Carbohydrate: 29 g
Fiber: 6 g
Net Carbohydrate: 23 g

### Uncle Sam Original Wheat Berry Flakes

Serving Size: ¾ cup
Calories: 210
Total Carbohydrate: 37 g
Fiber: 10 g
Net Carbohydrate: 27 g

## Breads

### Arnold Whole Grain Classic Bread

Serving Size: 1 slice
Calories: 100
Total Carbohydrate: 19 g
Fiber: 3 g
Net Carbohydrate: 16 g

### Doctor in the Kitchen Flackers

Serving Size: 8 crackers
Calories: 100
Total Carbohydrate: 7 g
Fiber: 6 g
Net Carbohydrate: 1 g

### GG Bran Crispbreads

Serving Size: 1 cracker
Calories: 20
Total Fat: 0 g
Total Carbohydrate: 6 g
Fiber: 4 g
Net Carbohydrate: 2 g

### La Tortilla Factory 100 calorie Tortilla

Serving Size: 1 tortilla
Calories: 100
Total Carbohydrate: 24 g
Fiber: 8 g
Net Carbohydrate: 16 g

### La Tortilla Whole Wheat Light Tortilla

Serving Size: 1 tortilla
Calories: 80
Total Carbohydrate: 16 g
Fiber: 8 g
Net Carbohydrate: 8 g

### Mission Carb Balance Tortilla (Fajita Size)

Serving Size: 1 tortilla
Calories: 80
Total Carbohydrate: 13 g
Fiber: 9 g
Net Carbohydrate: 4 g

### Nature's Own Life Wheat Double Fiber Bread

Serving Size: 1 slice
Calories: 50
Total Carbohydrate: 11 g
Fiber: 4 g
Net Carbohydrate: 7 g

### Publix Reduced Calorie, Natural Grain Bread

Serving Size: 2 slices

Calories: 90
Total Carbohydrate: 19 g
Fiber: 4 g
Net Carbohydrate: 15 g

**Thomas' English Muffins 100% Whole Wheat**
Serving Size: 1 muffin
Calories: 120
Total Carbohydrate: 22 g
Fiber: 3 g
Net Carbohydrate: 19 g

**Thomas' English Muffins Light Multigrain**
Serving Size: 1 muffin
Calories: 100
Total Carbohydrate: 25 g

Fiber: 8 g
Net Carbohydrate: 17 g

**Thomas' Mini Bagels 100% Whole Wheat**
Serving Size: 1 bagel
Calories: 110
Total Carbohydrate: 22 g
Fiber: 3 g
Net Carbohydrate: 19 g

**Wonder 100% Whole Wheat Bread**
Serving Size: 1 slice
Calories: 60
Total Carbohydrate: 11 g
Fiber: 2 g
Net Carbohydrate: 9 g

# INDEX

Agriculture Department, U.S., 7, 30, 133
alcoholic beverages, 131–33
American Dietetic Association, 5, 9, 71
appetite regulation, 169
appetizers, 140
Apple Cinnamon "Oatmeal," 184–85
Applesauce, Vanilla-Bean, 214–15
Arby's, 162
Asian Chicken Salad, 229
Asian Flavored Tuna, 212–13

Baer, David, 61
banana
  Chocolate Chip Muffins, 221–22
  Chocolate-Covered, 262–63
  Chunky Monkey F-Factor Smoothie, 219

Bard, Carl, 83
basal metabolic rate (BMR), 53–55
Baskin-Robbins, 162
beans, 34, 118
  Black, Salsa and Broiled Snapper, 248–49
  Black, Soup, 225–26
  and Grilled Beef Burgers, 242–43
  refried, 157
  Spiced Garbanzo, 234
  White, and Tuna Salad, 247–48
beef
  Best Meat Loaf, 243–44
  Classic Steak House Filet Mignon, 205
  Easy Fajitas, 240–41
  Grilled, and Bean Burgers, 242–43
  Grilled Sirloin Salad, 189–90
  step 1, 95

beef (*cont.*)
    TZ's Mozzarella-Stuffed
        Meatballs, 206–7
    Wholesome Sloppy Joes, 241–42
berry
    Breakfast Parfait, 181
    Cheesecake Parfait with
        Blackberry Sauce, 216–17
    Cranberry-Walnut Chutney, 261
    Crisp, 261–62
    Strawberry F-Factor Smoothie, 182
Best Meat Loaf, 243–44
Black Bean Soup, 225–26
Blackened Green Beans, 195
bloating, 79
blood lipids, 66–68
blood pressure, 69
Body Mass Index (BMI), 17, 19
body temperature, 169
bread, 32, 79, 116
    list of recommended, 273–74
breakfast
    benefits of, 93–94
    step 1, 98–99, 181–85
    step 2, 120–21, 124, 126,
        219–24
    step 3, 136
Breakfast Burritos, 220–21
breast cancer, 68–69
Broccoli Sesame Salad, 193
Broiled Baby Lamb Chops, 208
Broiled Salmon with Dill, 211–12
Broiled Snapper with Black Bean
    Salsa, 248–29
brown rice, 151
Brussels Sprouts, Roasted, 196
bulgur, 32, 117
    Tabouli Salad, 257–58

Burger King, 162
burgers
    Grilled Beef and Bean, 242–43
    Quinoa and Chickpea, in Lettuce
        Wraps, 256–57
    Southwest Turkey, 204
burritos
    Breakfast, 220–21
    Zesty Shrimp, 249–50
butyrate, 70

Cabbage Soup, 188
calories, 53–55
    in alcoholic drinks, 131–32
    burned in one hour, 170–71
    for weight loss, 55–56
carbohydrate groups, 31–37
    fruit/fruit juice list, 34–36,
        43–44, 118–20
    milk/yogurt list, 36–37, 44–45,
        120
    starch list, 32–34, 43, 116–18
carbohydrates, 12, 14
    adding to diet, 108–14, 135–36
    digestible amount of, 62–63
    do they make you fat?, 49–57
    grams per serving, 108
    high-fiber, 56–57, 129–30
    limiting, 85–86
carbo-loading, 52, 167
carbonated beverages, 105–6
cardiovascular disease, 66
cauliflower
    "Fried Rice," 232–33
    Pizza Crust, 197–98
celebrations, 144
cereal, 32–33, 116–17
    list of recommended, 271–73

cheese, 96
Cheesecake Parfait with Blackberry Sauce, 216–17
chicken
  Asian Salad, 229
  Crispy Pecan, 236–37
  Parmesan, Guiltless, 203–4
  Poached, Salad with Raspberry Vinaigrette, 201
  Ratatouille, 237–28
  Roasted, Harvest Bowl, 238–39
  Scallion and Ginger Spiced, 234–35
  Soup, 186
  Tandoori, 200
Chickpea and Quinoa Burgers in Lettuce Wraps, 256–57
Child, Julia, 177
Chili, Turkey, 239–40
Chinese Food, 150–51
Chips, Cinnamon Sugar Skinny, 260
chocolate, 141
  -Cherry-Almond Biscotti, 258–59
  Chip Banana Muffins, 221–22
  Chunky Monkey F-Factor Smoothie, 219
  -Covered Bananas, 262–63
cholesterol, 66
Chunky Monkey F-Factor Smoothie, 219
Cinnamon Sugar Skinny Chips, 260
Classic Steak House Filet Mignon, 205
colon cancer, 69–70
condiments, 97
constipation, 70–71, 73, 79–80
Corn Salsa, Roasted, 231–32
Crab Cakes, Maryland, 213–14

crackers, 33–34, 103, 118
Cranberry-Walnut Chutney, 261
Crispy Oven-Fried Fish, 246–47
Crispy Pecan Chicken, 236–37
Crispy Tilapia, 210–11
Crystal Light, 105

Dairy Queen, 162
dehydration, 129
desserts
  Cheesecake Parfait with Blackberry Sauce, 216–17
  Chocolate-Cherry-Almond Biscotti, 258–59
  Chocolate-Covered Bananas, 262–63
  Cranberry-Walnut Chutney, 261
  Grilled Fruit Kebabs, 217–18
  Macerated Fruit, 215–16
  step 1, 97, 214–18
diabetes, 66–68
dietician, 15–16
diets
  fad, 9–11
  high-fiber, 13–14
  high-protein, 56
  low-carb, 4–5
  low-fat, 4
  Mediterranean, 158
  problem with, 11
  very-low-calorie, 11
  without exercise, 167
dining out, 147–64
  Chinese food, 150–51
  fast food, 142–43, 161–64
  French food, 152–53
  Greek food, 158–59
  Indian food, 160–61

dining out (*cont.*)
   Italian food, 148–50
   Japanese food, 153–56
   Mexican food, 156–58
dinner
   step 1, 100–101
   step 2, 123–24, 128–29
   step 3, 136–37
*Dr. Atkins' Diet Revolution* (Atkins), 9
dried fruit, 140–41
drinks
   least caloric, 132
   most caloric, 132
   step 1, 97
Dunkin' Donuts, 162

Easy Beef Fajitas, 240–41
eating out. *See* dining out
Eggplant Rollatini, 193–95
eggs
   Greek Omelet, 183–84
   Italian Herb Frittata, 222–23
   Tuna Salad, 190
emotional eating, 168
energy
   caloric requirements, 53–55
   and high-fiber diet, 64
estrogen, 68
exchange lists, 31–42
exercise, 165–73
   benefits, 165, 167–69
   calories burned in one hour,
      170–71
   getting started, 169–70, 173
   weight training, 171–73

fad diets, 9–11
Fajitas, Easy Beef, 240–41

fast food, 142–43, 161–64
fasting, 56, 84
fat-free foods, 9–10
fat-free milk, 36
fat list, 41–42, 47
fats, 96
F-Factor Breakfast Sandwich,
   223–24
F-Factor Diet, 27–28
   development of, 12–13
   difference in, 12, 15
   and dining out. *See* dining out
   and exercise. *See* exercise
   mechanism of, 13–14
   overview of, 74–76
   recipes. *See* recipes
   steps in. *See* step 1; step 2; step 3
F-Factor's Famous High Fiber
   Pancake, 182–83
fiber, 12
   and blood pressure, 69
   boosting daily intake, 65
   and breast cancer, 68–69
   and colon cancer, 69–70
   and constipation, 70–71
   and diabetes, 66–68
   and energy, 64
   facts on, 60
   function of, 13
   GI tract adjustment to, 84
   goal for, 71
   and heart disease, 66
   insoluble (roughage), 60, 78
   in popular foods, 265–70
   soluble, 60
   sources of, 75–76
   from supplements, drinks, or
      pills, 73–74

Test Your Fiber IQ, 24–25
top ten myths about, 77–80
and weight loss, 56–57
what is it?, 59–60
fight-or-flight syndrome, 51
fish
    Asian Flavored Tuna, 212–13
    Broiled Salmon with Dill,
        211–12
    Broiled Snapper with Black Bean
        Salsa, 248–49
    Crispy Oven-Fried, 246–47
    Crispy Tilapia, 210–11
    step 1, 96
    Tuna and White Bean Salad,
        247–48
    Tuna-Egg Salad, 190
    See also shellfish
food
    fast, 142–43, 161–64
    fat-free, 9–10
    fiber content in popular, 265–70
    refined, 5–7
    step 1, 94–97
    step 2, 116–24
Food and Drug Administration, 7
food groups, 30–31
    four, 30
    six. See six food groups
food guide pyramid (USDA), 30–31
food labels, 109–12
four food groups, 30
Four Pepper Sauté, 199–200
French food, 152–53
frequently asked questions
    step 1, 103–6
    step 2, 129–33
    step 3, 142–44

"Fried Rice," Cauliflower, 232–33
fructose, 50
fruit, 34–35, 78, 118–19, 140–41
    Grilled Kebabs, 217–18
    Macerated, 215–16
fruit/fruit juice list, 34–36, 43–44,
    118–20
fruit juice, 32–33

Galileo Galilei, 49
game, 96
Garbanzo Beans, Spiced, 234
glucose, 50, 77, 167
glycemic index, 64
glycogen, 50
    depleting, 167
    storage of, 51–52
grains, 32–33, 116–17
    Nutty Stir-Fried Rice, 255–56
Greek food, 158–59
Greek Omelet, 183–84
Greek Salad, Lettuce-less, 230–31
Greek-Style Pork, 207
Greek yogurt, 104
Grilled Beef and Bean Burgers,
    242–43
Grilled Fruit Kebabs, 217–18
Grilled Sirloin Salad, 189–90
Grilled Veal Parmigiana, 208–9
Guiltless Chicken Parmesan, 203–4

Harvard School of Public Health,
    131
HDL cholesterol, 66
heart disease, 66
Heart Healthy Turkey Sausage, 185
high blood pressure, 69
high-fat meat/meat substitute list, 41

high-fiber diets, 13–14
high-protein diets, 56
holidays, 139–40, 144
Human Nutrition Research Center, 61
hypertension, 69

Indian food, 160–61
industrialization, 5–7
insoluble fiber (roughage), 60, 78
Italian food, 148–50
Italian Herb Frittata, 222–23

Japanese food, 153–56
journal
   step 1, 87–92, 102
   step 2, 114–15, 125
   step 3, 138, 145
*Journal of Clinical Oncology,* 68
*Journal of the American Medical Association,* 3, 61
*Joy of Cooking, The* (Rombauer and Becker), 8

Kebabs, Grilled Fruit, 217–18

lactose, 50
lamb
   Broiled Baby Chops, 208
   step 1, 95
Lao Tzu, 27
Lardner, Ring, 147
laxatives, 70–71
LDL cholesterol, 66
lean body mass, 172
Lean Cuisine Hearty Portions, 8–9
lean meat/meat substitute list, 39–40

lentils, 34, 118
   Moroccan Soup, 224–25
lettuce, 77–78
   Wraps, Quinoa and Chickpea Burgers in, 256–57
Lettuce-less Greek Salad, 230–31
Linguine with Clam Sauce, 254–55
liver, 53
low-carb diets, 4–5
low-fat diets, 4
low-fat milk, 36
lunch
   step 1, 99
   step 2, 121–22, 126–27
   step 3, 136
lycopene, 149

Macaroni and Cheese, 253–54
Macerated Fruit, 215–16
main dishes
   step 1
      beef, pork, and lamb, 205–9
      chicken and turkey, 200–204
      fish and shellfish, 209–14
   step 2
      beef, pork, and lamb, 240–46
      chicken and turkey, 234–40
      fish and shellfish, 246–52
      pasta and grains, 252–58
maintenance. *See* step 3
maltose, 50
Maryland Crab Cakes, 213–14
McDonald's, 7, 162, 164
Meatballs, TZ's Mozzarella-Stuffed, 206–7
meat loaf
   Best, 243–44
   Turkey, 202

meat/meat substitute list, 46–47
  high-fat meat, 41
  lean meat, 39–40
  medium-fat meat, 40
  very-lean meat, 38–39
Mediterranean diet, 158
mental health, 168
menu plan
  step 1, 101–3
  step 2, 124–26
  step 3, 136–37, 138
metabolism, 53–55, 130, 167–68
Metamucil, 73
Mexican food, 156–58
midday munchies, 137–39
milk/yogurt list, 36–37, 44–45, 120
Minestrone Soup, 226–27
monounsaturated fat, 41–42, 47
Moroccan Lentil Soup, 224–25
Muffins, Banana Chocolate Chip,
  221–22
multivitamins, 104–5
muscles, 50–51, 53, 172
myths
  about carbs, 49–57
  about fiber, 77–80

National Academy of Sciences, 71,
  154
National Institute of Public Health, 4
National Restaurant Association, 8,
  147
National Weight Loss Registry, 93
non-carbohydrate groups, 31,
  37–42, 45–47
nondieters, 141–42
nonstarchy vegetables list, 37–38,
  45–46

nutrition
  education, 15
  exchange lists, 31–42
  facts labels, 114
  food groups. *See* food groups
  Quiz: Carbohydrate, Protein, or
    Fat?, 29
nuts, 96
Nutty Stir-Fried Rice, 255–56

"Oatmeal," Apple Cinnamon, 184–85
Oats, Pumpkin Spice Overnight,
  219–20
obesity, 3, 162
  and fad diets, 9–11
  and industrialization, 5–7
  and portion sizes, 7–9
omega-3 fatty acids, 154
omelets. *See* eggs
overweight vs. obese, 17

Pancakes, F-Factor's Famous High-
  Fiber, 182–83
parfait
  Berry Breakfast, 181
  Cheesecake, with Blackberry
    Sauce, 216–17
pasta, 148
  Bolognese, 252–53
  Linguine with Clam Sauce,
    254–55
  Macaroni and Cheese, 253–54
peas, 34, 118
*Pediatrics,* 68–69
Pepper, Four, Sauté, 199–200
Percival, Lord, 165
phyllo, 158
Pizza Crust, Cauliflower, 197–98

Poached Chicken Salad with
  Raspberry Vinaigrette, 201
polyunsaturated fat, 42, 47
pork
  Greek-Style, 207
  step 1, 95
portion sizes, 7–9, 152
poultry, 95
  *See also* chicken; turkey
protein, 13, 86–88
Pumpkin Spice Overnight Oats,
  219–20

Quinoa and Chickpea Burgers in
  Lettuce Wraps, 256–57

recipes, 177–263
  step 1, 179
    beef, pork, and lamb main
      dishes, 205–9
    breakfast, 181–85
    chicken and turkey main dishes,
      200–204
    desserts, 214–18
    fish and shellfish main dishes,
      209–14
    soup, salad, and sides, 186–200
  steps 2 and 3, 180
    beef, pork, and lamb main
      dishes, 240–46
    breakfast, 219–24
    chicken and turkey main dishes,
      234–40
    desserts, 258–63
    fish and shellfish main dishes,
      246–52
    pasta and grains, 252–58
    soups, salads, and sides, 224–34

reduced-fat milk, 36
refined foods, 5–7
refried beans, 157
restaurants. *See* dining out
resting metabolic rate (RMR),
  167–68
Rice, Nutty Stir-Fried, 255–56
Roasted Brussels Sprouts, 196
Roasted Chicken Harvest Bowl,
  238–39
Roasted Corn Salsa, 231–32
Rockefeller, John D., 107
roughage, 60, 78

salads, 77–78
  Asian Chicken, 229
  Broccoli Sesame, 193
  Grilled Sirloin, 189–90
  Lettuce-less Greek, 230–31
  Poached Chicken, with Raspberry
    Vinaigrette, 201
  Spinach with Warm Bacon
    Vinaigrette, 191
  Tabouli, 257–58
  Tanya's House, 228
  Tuna and White Bean, 247–48
  Tuna-Egg, 190
Salmon, Broiled, with Dill, 211–12
Salsa, Roasted Corn, 231–32
Sandwich, F-Factor Breakfast,
  223–24
sashimi, 153–54
satiety, 13
saturated fat, 42, 47
sauces, 152, 155
Sausage, Heart Healthy Turkey, 185
Scallion and Ginger Spiced
  Chicken, 234–35

seasonings, 97
shellfish
    Maryland Crab Cakes, 213–14
    Shrimp with Feta Cheese, 209–10
    step 1, 96
    Thai Shrimp Summer Rolls,
        251–52
    Zesty Shrimp Burritos, 249–50
shopping list, 85
shrimp
    Burritos, Zesty, 249–50
    with Feta Cheese, 209–10
    Summer Rolls, Thai, 251–52
side dishes
    Blackened Green Beans, 195
    Eggplant Rollatini, 193–95
    Four Pepper Sauté, 199–200
    Roasted Brussels Sprouts, 196
    Sautéed Zucchini with Parmesan,
        198–99
    Spiced Garbanzo Beans, 234
    String Beans in Tomato Sauce,
        192
    Sweet Potato Chips, 233
six food groups, 30–31
    fats, 41–42, 47
    fruit/fruit juice, 34–36, 43–44
    meat/meat substitutes, 38–41,
        46–47
    milk/yogurt, 36–37, 44–45
    nonstarchy vegetables, 37–38,
        45–46
    starches, 32–34, 43
skipping meals, 84, 92–94
Sloppy Joes, Wholesome, 241–42
smoothies
    Chunky Monkey F-Factor, 219
    Strawberry F-Factor, 182

snacks
    afternoon, 137–39
    healthy, 139
    step 1, 33–34
    step 2, 118, 122–23, 127–28
    step 3, 136
Snapper, Broiled, with Black Bean
        Salsa, 248–49
Socrates, 3
soluble fiber, 60
soups
    Black Bean, 225–26
    Cabbage, 188
    Chicken, 186
    Minestrone, 226–27
    Moroccan Lentil, 224–25
    Vegetable, 187–88
Southwest Turkey Burgers, 204
Spiced Garbanzo Beans, 234
Spinach Salad with Warm Bacon
        Vinaigrette, 191
Starbucks, 7
starch list, 32–34, 43, 116–18
starchy vegetables, 33, 117
starvation mode, 56, 84, 130
statins, 66
step 1, 74, 83–106
    benefits, 84
    breakfast, 98–99
    carbohydrates allowed, 85–86
    dinner, 100–101
    foods allowed, 94–97
    foods to avoid, 97–98
    frequently asked questions, 103–6
    journal for, 87–92, 102
    lunch, 99
    no skipping meals/snacks, 92–93
    other requirements, 103

step 1 (*cont.*)
  protein guidelines, 86, 87
  recipes, 179
    breakfast, 181–85
    desserts, 214–18
    main dishes, 200–214
    soup, salad, and sides, 186–200
  sample menu and journal entry,
    101–3
  shopping list, 85
  snacks, 33–34
step 2, 74–76, 107–33
  adding carbs, 108–9
  benefits, 107–8
  breakfast, 120–21, 124
    tips for, 126
  carbs per serving, 108
  dinner, 123–24
    tips for, 128–29
  foods allowed, 116–24
  frequently asked questions,
    129–33
  journal for, 114–15, 125
  lunch, 121–22
    tips for, 126–27
  recipes, 180
    breakfast, 219–24
    desserts, 258–63
    main dishes, 234–58
    soup, salad, and sides,
     224–34
  sample daily menu, 72–73
  sample menu and journal entry,
    124–26
  snacks, 118, 122–23
    tips for, 127–28
  time to stay on, 114
step 3, 76, 135–45

  adding three more carb servings,
    135–36
  breakfast, 136
  dinner, 136–37
  frequently asked questions,
    142–44
  lunch, 136
  sample menu and journal entry,
    136–37, 138, 145
  snacks, 136
  staying motivated, 137
    eating with nondieters, 141–42
    holidays, 139–40
    midday munchies, 137–39
    sweets cravings, 140–41
Strawberry F-Factor Smoothie,
  182
String Beans in Tomato Sauce, 192
Subway, 162
sugar, 50
Summer Rolls, Thai Shrimp,
  251–52
supermarket, 80
supplements
  fiber, 73–74, 78
  multivitamin, 104–5
sushi, 153–54
Sweet Potato Chips, 233
sweet treats, 140–41

Tabouli Salad, 257–58
Tandoori Chicken, 200
Tanya's House Salad, 228
technology, 6
tempura, 155
Thai Shrimp Summer Rolls,
  251–52
Tilapia, Crispy, 210–11

tuna
  Asian Flavored, 212–13
  -Egg Salad, 190
  and White Bean Salad, 247–48
turkey
  Chili, 239–40
  Meat Loaf, 202
  Sausage, Heart Healthy, 185
  Southwest Burgers, 204
  TZ's Mozzarella-Stuffed Meatballs,
    206–7

University of Massachusets, 93

vacations, 144
Vanderbilt University, 93
Vanilla-Bean Applesauce,
  214–15
veal
  Grilled Parmigiana, 208–9
  step 1, 95
vegetables, 78
  step 1, 95
vegetable side dishes. See side
  dishes

Vegetable Soup, 187–88
very lean meat/meat substitute list,
  38–39
very-low-calorie diets, 11

water, 105, 128–29
weight, 166
weight loss
  and calories, 55–56
  and fiber, 56–57
  jump-starting, 83–84
weight training, 168, 171–73
Welles, Orson, 135
Wendy's, 162
white rice, 151
whole grains, 5
whole milk, 37
Wholesome Sloppy Joes, 241–42

yogurt, 104

Zesty Shrimp Burritos, 249
zucchini
  Noodle Bolognese, 244–46
  Sautéed, with Parmesan, 198–99

# ABOUT THE AUTHOR

TANYA ZUCKERBROT, M.S., R.D., is a nutritionist and the creator of the F-Factor diet, which she has used for more than twenty years to provide thousands of clients with all the tools they need to achieve easy weight loss and maintenance and improved health and well-being. F-Factor is the leading dietitian-created program for weight loss and optimal health based upon fiber-rich nutrition that helps people effectively and positively improve their lives without disrupting their lifestyle.

Tanya has appeared on the *View*, the *Today Show*, the *Early Show*, the *Rachael Ray Show*, MSNBC, *ABC News*, *Good Morning America Health*, *CBS Evening News*, *Extra*, *Good Day New York*, and on many other local and national media platforms. She is a nutrition news contributor for the Fox News Channel and writes a weekly column for Foxnews.com. She has been profiled in the *New York Times*, and has been featured in the *New York Post*, the *New York Daily News*, *Town & Country*, *Elle*, *Vogue*, *Allure*, *Self*, the *Huffington Post*, the *Miami Herald*, the *Washington Post*, and the *Daily Mail*.

In addition, Tanya is an international speaker and spokesperson. She has lectured for NBC Studios, the Discovery Network, Procter & Gamble, Johnson & Johnson, G&E, and Estée Lauder. Most recently Tanya became a brand ambassador for the retailer Saks Fifth Avenue.

Tanya holds a master's degree in nutrition and food studies from New York University and completed a two-year dietetic internship at the NYU Medical Center. She is an accredited member of the American Dietetic Association, the Greater New York Dietetic Association, and a member of the National Association of Professional Women. Tanya completed her CDR Certificate of Training in Adult Weight Management as well as her CDR Certificate of Training in Childhood and Adolescent Weight Management. Tanya is a Medical Advisory Board Member of Sharsheret.

She is the author of two bestselling weight loss books: *The F-Factor Diet: Discover the Secret to Permanent Weight Loss*, and *The Miracle Carb Diet: Make Calories and Fat Disappear the F-Factor Way—with Fiber!*

Tanya resides in New York City with her husband and their children.